S THE ART OF *Sensual* Aromatherapy

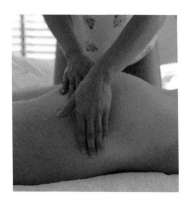

Henry Holt and Company, Inc.
Publishers since 1866
115 West 18th Street
New York, New York 10011

Henry Holt® is a registered trademark of Henry Holt
and Company, Inc.

Library of Congress Catalog Card Number: 95-77886

ISBN 0-8050-4153-2

Henry Holt books are available for special
promotions and premiums. For details contact:
Director, Special Markets.

First Edition—1995

Executive Editor: Lorraine Dickey
Art Direction and design: Zoë Maggs
Photographer: Susanna Price
Picture Research: Charlotte Bush
Project Editors: Nicky Hodge, Sarah Larter
Production: Sarah Schuman

Printed and bound in Great Britain
All first editions are printed on acid-free paper. ∞

10 9 8 7 6 5 4 3 2 1

Thanks to Applewoods International Limited, Devon,
England for the use of their Aromatherapy oils.

The information contained in this book is not meant
as a replacement for diagnosis or treatment by a
qualified medical practitioner. In regard to the
essential oils and massage, all information and
recommendations are believed to be true but as the
authors are unable to monitor the quality or
appropriate use of massage or the essential oils, no
expressed nor implied guarantee as to the effects of
their use can be given. The author and publisher
disclaim all responsibility for adverse reactions and
accept no liability. If in doubt, always seek the
advice of a doctor.

The publishers would like to thank the following
sources for their kind permission to reproduce the
pictures in this book:

A-Z Botanical; Pat Brindley; Neil Campbell-Sharp;
Royal Botanic Garden, Edinburgh; Royal Horticultural
Society; The Harry Smith Horticultural Photographic
Collection; Sunspirit Oils Ltd; Elizabeth Whiting
Associates.

Every effort has been made to acknowledge correctly
and contact the source and/or copyright holder of
each picture, and Carlton Books Limited apologises
for any unintentional errors or omissions which will
be corrected in future editions of this book.

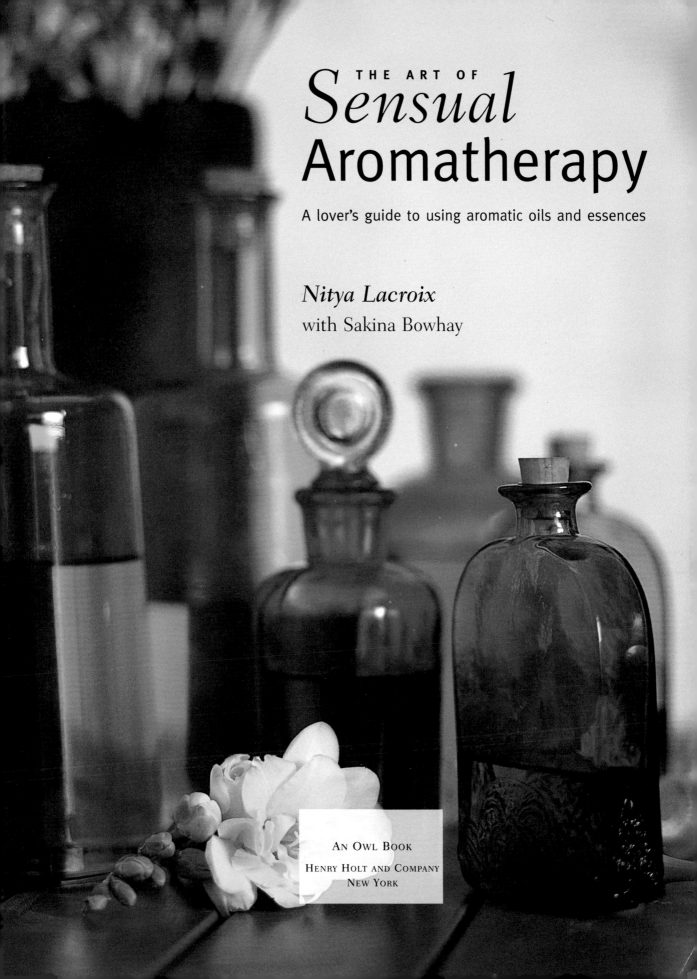

THE ART OF
Sensual
Aromatherapy

A lover's guide to using aromatic oils and essences

Nitya Lacroix

with Sakina Bowhay

AN OWL BOOK
HENRY HOLT AND COMPANY
NEW YORK

CONTENTS

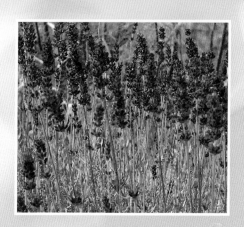
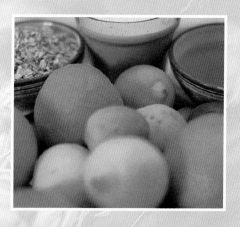
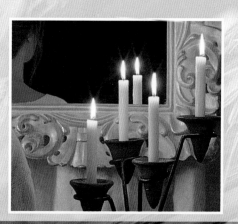

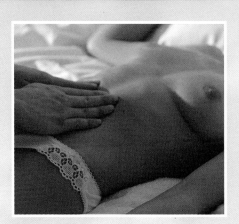
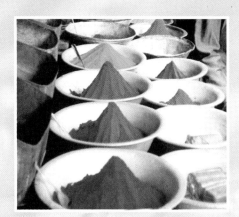
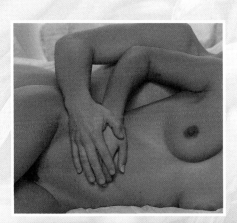

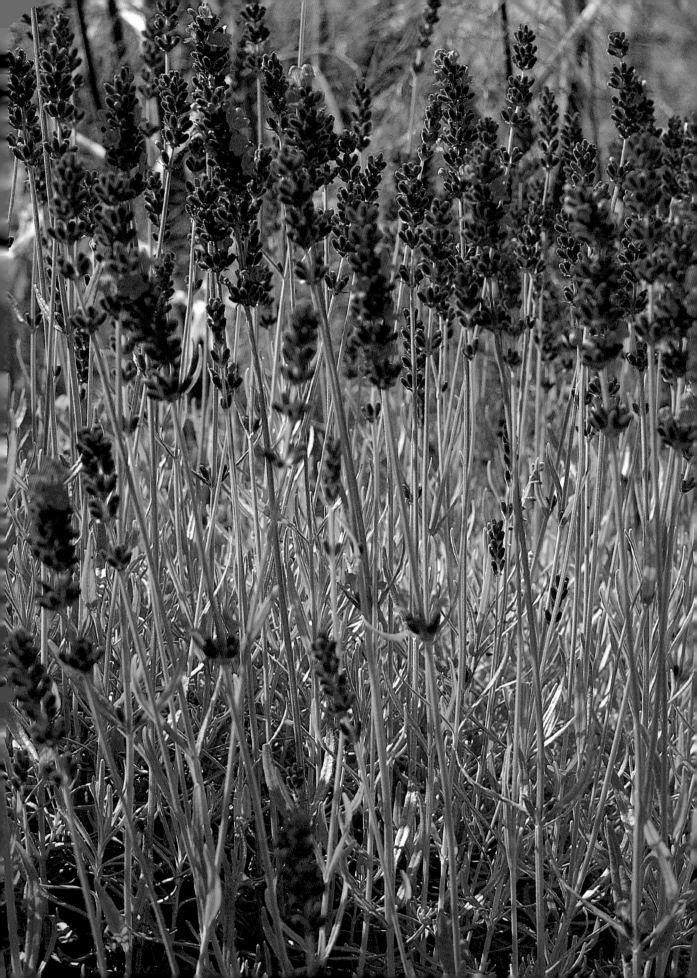

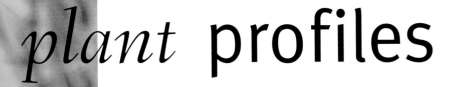

plant profiles

Essential oils are the gifts of nature and have been treasured by humankind since ancient times. These aromatic essences enhance all aspects of life, whether they are used to soothe and heal the mind and body, to beautify the skin, to increase sensuality and feelings of pleasure, or to elevate spiritual consciousness. Their fragrances are drawn from fruits, flowers, herbs, spices, and the woods of trees by different methods of distillation. By using them according to instruction, it is possible to invite into your home the smells of the forest, the bright sunshine cheer of the citrus grove, the exotic perfumes of the East, the pungent odors of a spice market, and the herbaceous scents of a country garden.

The aromatic oils are a feast for our senses, and their individual properties work their magic in a holistic way on every aspect of body, mind, and soul. In this book, we have selected eighteen of the oils for the reader to come to know and love, and they have been chosen specifically for their sensual and aphrodisiac enhancement or their emotionally evocative properties. They are selected especially for lovers to bring beauty and enjoyment into the lives of all who wish to celebrate the joy of sensuality, and the ecstasy of erotic love. At the same time, their nurturing properties will help to release physical and emotional tensions.

BASIL
(Ocimum Basilium)

Erotic

The herb basil has a sweet, spicy aroma, with a hint of camphor, and has many associations with love, seduction, and fertility. As an aphrodisiac essence, basil has gained a reputation for awakening the senses and arousing the most basic sexual instincts – it was used by young Italian women to charm and bewitch the men of their desires. Indeed basil, which is best known for its culinary uses, was added to food whenever it was deemed that the enticing powers of Venus, the love goddess, were failing to exact the required results.

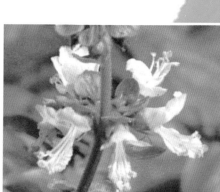

Basil's essential oil, extracted from the shrub's leaves and flowering tops, can be used to reawaken a sexual relationship that has waned in intensity or interest, or when someone is anxious or lacks experience. Some say that its name comes from basileus, the Greek for "king" because its wonderful smell is fit for royalty. Basil originates from India where myth has it that the Hindu gods, Krishna and Vishnu, bestowed upon it protective and inspirational properties. It now grows extensively around the world, most notably across southern Europe, North Africa, Java, the Seychelles, and North America.

Basil's strengthening, stimulating and restorative properties help to ease mental, emotional, and physical fatigue and, when added to a base oil and rubbed into the body, remove weariness from tense, tired muscles. Its restorative properties are said to ease headaches, respiratory infections, sinus problems, asthma, and flu.

Caution: Avoid use during pregnancy. Apply with care on sensitive skin.

BERGAMOT

(*Citrus Bergamia*)

Evocative

When added to a blend of aphrodisiac oils, bergamot's uplifting, enticing, and refreshing properties can greatly enhance the sensual mood of lovers. Whether it is used in an aromatic burner, or blended with oils to be used in a massage, its delightful lemon and floral aroma will do much to lift and balance a loved one's spirit. Adding the component of happiness and contentment to a blend – bergamot is indeed a gift to any relationship.

The essence from bergamot is commonly used in perfumes; this is what gives Earl Grey tea its distinctive flavor. It was once much favored as a perfume for spices and floral decorations, especially at times of celebration such as marriage ceremonies or to welcome a baby's birth.

Bergamot comes from a small tree that grows mainly in Italy and some parts of Africa. The essence is expressed from the rind of its unusual citrus fruit. It can be used whenever a partner is anxious or depressed, or prone to heated outbursts of temper, as it is able to help alleviate tension and anxiety. Bergamot cools feverish conditions and has been used in the treatment of urinary tract infections such as cystitis – it can also soothe the digestive and respiratory system, encouraging appetite and a return to health during convalescence.

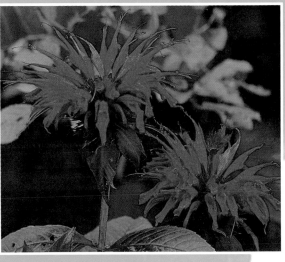

Caution: Do not apply to skin to be exposed to sunlight or ultraviolet light; it increases the skin's photosensitivity. It may irritate sensitive skin.

BLACK PEPPER
(Piper nigrum)

Erotic

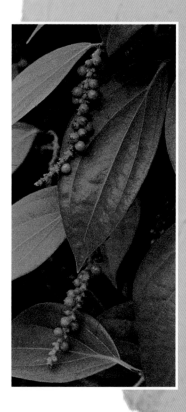

Black pepper adds spice and vitality to a love life. With its warming, penetrating, and strengthening properties, black pepper has earned itself a reputation as an aphrodisiac. Its amber oil extract is used to rekindle the flame of passion when a relationship has cooled either from lack of interest or familiarity. Emitting a sharp, spicy aroma that arouses the senses and supplies the stamina and strength, black pepper warms up not only the body, but also the emotions, revitalizing and enhancing a loving encounter.

Records of black pepper's uses as an aphrodisiac have been made throughout history. Ancient Arabic manuals giving advice on sexual matters refer to its erotic properties. In Roman times, it was liberally used, not only as a spice for cooking, but to add strength and stamina to a man's performance, both on the battlefield and in the bedroom. During the bathing rituals of the Roman era – often a prelude to a night of hedonistic pleasure – servants added the essence of black pepper to oils which they used to anoint their masters' bodies.

The essential oil of black pepper is distilled from the plant's red berries that are picked before they ripen and dried naturally in the sun. In ancient times, black pepper was so highly regarded as a spice that battles were fought over it, and it was sometimes traded, ounce for ounce, for the same price as gold.

A stimulating essential oil that can warm and ease stiffness in cold, tense muscles and increase their tone, black pepper's spicy properties can also refresh the mind and help to banish fatigue.

Caution: Black pepper's essential oil may irritate some skins.

CEDARWOOD

(Cedrus atlantica/Juniperus virginiana)

Evocative

The essence of cedarwood is a profoundly evocative oil when used to open up the emotions, helping lovers to enter into the spirit of the here-and-now in lovemaking, which can give their physical union a more spiritual dimension. Soothing fears and anxieties associated with sexuality, this essence encourages lovers to let go of their emotions in lovemaking by drawing them into the blissful and sensual reality of the present moment.

The cedar is a beautiful and majestic coniferous evergreen tree. The essential oil that is distilled from its wood has been revered since ancient times for its relaxing and meditative qualities. The cedar tree is frequently mentioned in the Bible, often in relation to fertility. In many parts of the world, it has been known as the "tree of life" or the "tree of gods", being renowned as a symbol of faith and strength.

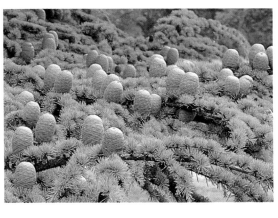

Varying species of cedar grow throughout the world's regions, but it is the *Cedrus Atlantica* that is most often preferred in the use of aromatherapy. It is also commonly used in incense, to perfume the home as well as during religious ceremonies.

Cedarwood's dry, woody aroma can soothe an anxious mind. Its properties help to alleviate many physical complaints and work well on the respiratory system. Its soothing qualities are used in skincare to preserve youthful beauty. Cedarwood essential oil can help relieve irritated skin or an itchy scalp and is particularly good for oily skin.

Caution: Do not use during pregnancy.

CLARY SAGE
(Salvia sclarea)

Erotic

Euphoric is the word most commonly associated with clary sage. A deeply sensual oil, reputed to have aphrodisiac qualities, clary sage has relaxing and calming properties that can decrease inhibitions. It is a helpful essential oil, particularly in boosting libido whenever either one or both partners are under stress and have external worries standing in the way of sexual ease. It helps to dissolve fears

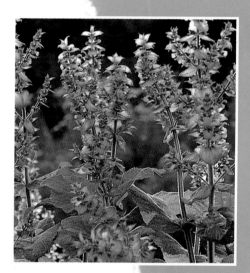

and anxieties that create the emotional blocks at the root of sexual dysfunction, and thus enables partners to enter a deeper, more intimate and trusting communication.

Clary sage has a strong, dry, and nutty aroma, which can produce a sense of mild intoxication, capable of adding a touch of wild and gay abandon to a night of lovemaking. Clary sage encourages creative thought, but because it can also be very soporific, it is best used for times of pleasure and relaxation. Clary sage should not be used before driving or any function requiring focused concentration.

In the past, clary sage's mildly intoxicating qualities were used in white magic spells to ignite the interest of a desired lover. Certainly, its essence, when mixed with other oils, adds greatly to the sensuality of a body massage when used as a prelude to making love.

Clary sage is grown in many countries and its oil is distilled from its flowering tops and leaves. It is an aid in the treatment of digestive, respiratory, and stress-related female reproductive disorders.

Caution: Do not use in combination with alcohol or in any large doses, as it can cause nausea. Clary sage should not be used in pregnancy, or by women who experience heavy menstrual flow.

FRANKINCENSE
(*Boswellia carteri*)

Evocative

The haunting, resinous aroma of frankincense brings depth and meaning to a relationship, for this meditative and fortifying essence will elevate personal and spiritual love. Heightening awareness on all levels, frankincense can help those who seek inner peace and a realization of their truth. Used within a relationship, it will enhance communication between the two people.

Since time immemorial, frankincense has been used to inspire and awaken the spiritual senses. Burned, or used as incense, in churches, temples, or places of worship, frankincense's haunting fragrance was thought to ascend to the heavens and perfume paradise. Noted for its quality of transformation, expanding consciousness, and imbuing the mind with calm and peace, this essence is used to enhance both contemplation and exaltation.

Used within the home, the aroma from frankincense can stimulate the senses, nourish the spirit, comfort the mind, and integrate the emotions. Like cedarwood, it has the quality of the here and now, drawing body and mind into the present moment of blissful repose.

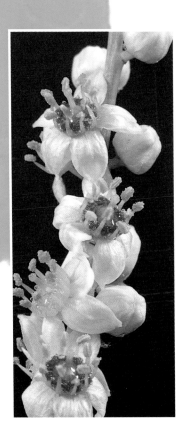

Frankincense is distilled from a resinous gum that exudes from a small and leafy deciduous tree originating from the Middle East – it is now also found in North Africa. It benefits the physical body, and assists the respiratory and digestive system. It was used by Egyptian women both in kohl for their eyes and as a rejuvenating cosmetic. It helps to preserve a youthful skin and, in combination with other oils, is particularly beneficial to mature and oily skin.

There are no known precautions.

GINGER
(*Zingiber officinalis*)

Erotic

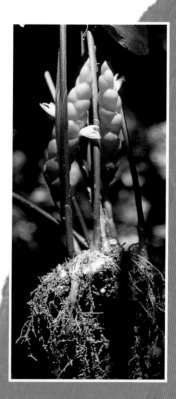

Pungent and spicy, a touch of ginger essence will boost and add vitality to a love relationship, bringing to it a warmth to melt cold emotions and a sizzle to heat up the libido.

Ginger has long been used for its culinary and medical properties, but its reputation as an aphrodisiac seems to be as equally established. The Romans certainly made use of its sexually enhancing properties, adding it to a mulled wine mixed with cinnamon, rhubarb, and vanilla to inflame the passions of desire at special festivals and celebrations. Avicenna, the great Roman physician and philosopher, who is credited with inventing the process of distillation, extolled the virtues of ginger mixed with honey as a curative for male impotence. He stated that it would increase the blood circulation to the penis and ensure a manly erection. An old Turkish recipe said much the same, advising couples to blend ginger and honey in a concoction to drink at night to inflame desire and increase fertility. Ginger, needless to say, was a spice despised by English Puritans, who feared it would provoke "unseemly passion."

The ginger plant originated in Asia and flourishes in moist, warm climates. It was one of the earliest spices to find its way to Europe through the ancient spice trade route. The essential oil is distilled from the root of the plant – its properties are invigorating and warming, which can help to boost blood circulation. It is a very stimulating oil for all the vital resources of the body. When added to a massage blend, ginger will warm and loosen stiff muscles.

Caution: Ginger can irritate a sensitive skin.

G E R A N I U M

(Pelargonium graveloens/
Pelargonium odoratissimum)

Evocative

This popular and lovely plant has a special place in the hearts of many people, for its brightly colored flowers cheer the eye on many windowsills and balconies throughout the world. Although these plants are commonly known as geraniums, their proper name is pelargoniums. Its essence brings a sense of equilibrium to a relationship, for its properties have the closest yin-and-yang balance of all the essential oils – the principle in which all opposing universal polarities can unite in perfect harmony. Thus geranium can help to integrate the essential differences of male and female energy, enabling a loving couple to reach a greater mutual understanding.

The essence of geranium neither stimulates nor relaxes, but adds a sustaining and restoring quality of well-being to any blend of oils. Added to a massage oil, a bath, or to an aromatic burner, geranium will imbue the atmosphere with its rich floral perfume, helping a couple to communicate and resolve issues that concern them both. Like the rose, the plant is said to be ruled by Venus, the Goddess of Love.

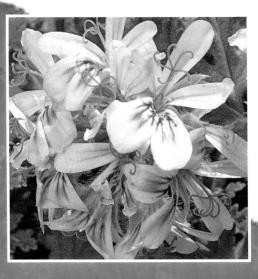

Only a few species of geranium are cultivated for their essential oil. Geranium essence is used frequently in perfumes and soaps, being a good addition to skincare as it suits all skin types. A tonic to the body's circulatory system, it works well in balancing the hormonal system.

Geranium has no known precautions, but people with sensitive skins should exercise caution when adding this essential oil to bathwater.

JASMINE ABSOLUTE

*(Jasminium officinalis/
Jasminium grandiflorum)*

Erotic

The heady and exotic perfume from the white, star-shaped flowers of jasmine has an equally seductive appeal to both men and women. Known as the "king of flowers," this romantic plant exudes its exquisite aroma mostly at night and must be picked before the morning dew to gain its full therapeutic value as an essential oil.

Jasmine is steeped in history as an aphrodisiac and a plant of love, having been used since ancient times in potions and spells to capture, sustain, or rekindle the affection of a loved one. A fragrant emblem of love, it promises deep and lasting affection and is entwined among the bridal flowers at Indian weddings – the wreath being a symbolic bond that eternally unites the bridal couple. In India, its ghostly pale flowers have earned jasmine the name "moonlight of the grove". One ancient Indian myth tells the story

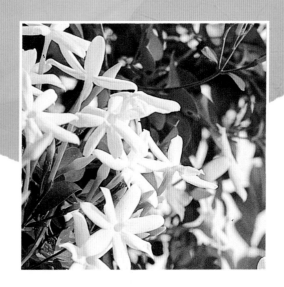

of a beautiful princess who fell in love with Surya-Deva, the sun god. Heartbroken by his rejection, she killed herself, but where her ashes were scattered, there grew the beautiful jasmine bush. Since the sun god was responsible for the princess' death, the jasmine will only release its heavenly perfume at night. Jasmine originates from Asia, where it was deemed a sacred flower. The sensual character of jasmine's oil brings strength and warmth to a sexual relationship. Jasmine can be added to massage oil to boost confidence and reduce lethargy, and relax muscles and joints.

Caution: Jasmine should not be used during pregnancy.

JUNIPER
(*Juniperus communis*)

Erotic

Juniper is the plant of protection, cleansing negative feelings of past

relationships and providing the strength, courage, and support to form a new one. Its stimulating properties are well known as an aphrodisiac – in olden times it was added to potions and recipes to awaken love and sexuality, as well as providing a protection from diseases of the devil. Juniper essential oil can be used whenever someone is feeling insecure and unworthy of love, strengthening resolve and providing protection while trust is still to be formed within a new relationship.

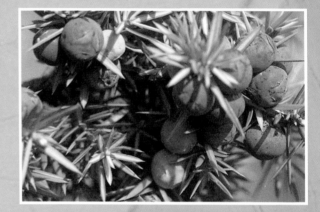

The essential oil is obtained from the ripe, blue juniper berries, which are also an important ingredient in gin giving it its distinctive flavor. Its aroma blends well with other oils.

Juniper has been used throughout the ages as a spiritual and bodily protector. In Britain, juniper was once hung on the front doors of houses to keep away witches on the eve of May, and its wood was frequently burned to banish demons.

The essential oil can help to clear a burdened mind, building up emotional reserves especially when someone has given too much of themselves to love. An excellent diuretic, juniper can help to cleanse the body of toxins and speed recovery in convalescence. It can act as a sedative when used in small doses, and as a stimulant when the dosage is increased.

Caution: Do not use if pregnant or if suffering from kidney disease.

LAVENDER
(Lavendula officinalis)

Evocative

Lavender has a special beauty of its own. Few things are more lovely than the sight of its purple-blue flowers nodding in the breeze on a sunny day, while its clear, light, and flowery fragrance fills the air with a distinctive aroma.

While lavender essential oil is not an aphrodisiac stimulant in its own right, it is soothing to the heart, and its relaxing and balancing properties mean that many people include it when preparing recipes for lovemaking. Lavender is also a popular ingredient in pot pourri and scents for the bedroom, especially to those who appreci-

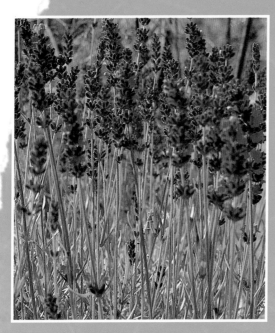

ate its comforting aroma. With healing and nurturing qualities that bring calm and peace to a relationship, this essence can expand and soothe the mind, creating a sense of timelessness within which lovers can enjoy a deep and gentle meeting with each other.

Lavender is one of the most used essential oils in aromatherapy because of the diversity of its nature and its ability to blend well.

The essential oil is distilled from the leaves, flowers, and stems of the plant. The Pharaohs of Egypt used it as a fragrance, and the Romans bathed in lavender water. It works well as an analgesic, easing muscular pain and tension, soothing cuts, scratches, and burns. Excellent for skincare, it suits all skin types and promotes the generation of healthy new tissue.

Caution: Do not use during the first three months of pregnancy.

LIME

(Citrus acris/Citrus aurantifolia)

Evocative

A few drops of lime in a lovers' blend of essential oils will add cheer

and laughter to a romance, whetting the appetite for desire and passion and filling the atmosphere with a sense of joy and lightness. For those who are taking themselves too seriously, it will enhance the feeling of childlike playfulness and fun. Lime's essential oil lifts the spirits and eases anxiety, relieving the mind of small, petty, and repetitious thoughts, to clear a pathway for lovers' communication.

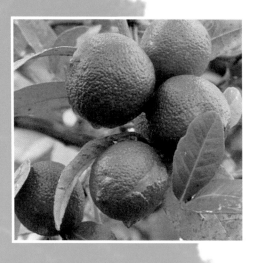

Lime has a sharp, sweet, mouthwatering citrus aroma, which is refreshing to both the mind and body, boosting energy when resources are low. Its essential oil is expressed from the rind of its fruit, which is green in color though sometimes tinged with yellow.

Lime blossom is a symbol of undying and eternal love. When Baucis and Philemon asked the great god, Zeus, to unite them after death, he turned them into two lime trees that grew side by side. This story is reflected in many literary legends that describe a perfect marriage as the growth of two lime trees standing side by side, bringing forth flowers and fruit, yet never in each others' shadow.

Mixed into an oil blend and rubbed into the body, lime provides an excellent digestive stimulant and can be used in convalescence to encourage a healthy appetite. Lime tones and refreshes the skin and is of particular benefit to oily skin.

Caution: This essential oil may cause photosensitivity to sunlight and can possibly irritate sensitive skin.

NEROLI ABSOLUTE

(Citrus aurantium/citrus vulgaris)

Erotic

Orange blossom, from which neroli's essential oil is distilled, has come to symbolize both seduction and sexual purity throughout its long history of aromatic use. Orange blossom was woven into a bride's floral bouquet for hundreds of years to guarantee not only good luck and happiness, but also fertility. Any bride who wore orange blossom in her hair did so to proclaim her virginity. Yet, several centuries ago, neroli's haunting, bitter sweet perfume was used by Madrid's "women of the night" to seduce and lure their clients.

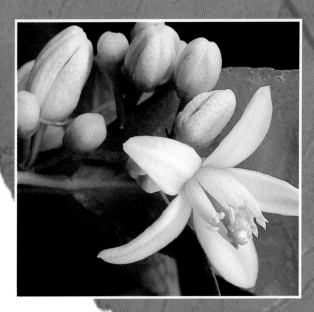

While neroli comes from the bitter Seville orange tree, the name is derived from the title of an Italian princess, Anne-Marie of Nerola, who used the perfume to fragrance her gloves and bathing water. Many noble women followed suit; it was also renowned for its use as a perfume in the court of Queen Elizabeth I of England. Neroli also has a history of use in aphrodisiac potions, specifically to aid virility. One Arabic recipe recommended it as a cure for impotence. Neroli evokes the sense of contentment. Acting as both an aphrodisiac and a relaxant in times of anxiety-related sexual problems, it will ease communication, enabling partners to reach deeper clarity. It is a general tonic for the whole system and is useful when someone is in a state of shock.

There are no known precautions.

O R A N G E
(Citrus vulgaris/Citrus aurantium)

Evocative

Like many of the citric essential oils, orange brings cheerful warmth as well as the sunshine and brightness of its native lands into the lives of lovers. Encouraging a mood of joy and sensuality, the essential oil adds pep and zest to a long-term partnership that may have become tinged with boredom. Its sweet, warm citric aroma will put vitality back into lovemaking.

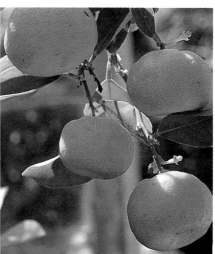

Orange and neroli share a common history, the essence of orange coming from the fruit of the tree and neroli from its blossoms. The tree originates from China, but now also grows in France, Portugal, the Americas, and the Mediterranean lands.

According to mythology, the orange is the "golden apple," the fruit given to Juniper by Juno on the day of their celestial wedding. In folklore, the exchange of an orange as a gift between an unmarried boy and girl is a simple charm that invites love between the two. In many legends, it is the fruit of seduction – certainly one forever associated with Nell Gwynn, the orange seller who won the heart of an English king. Oranges are also symbols of fertility.

It is a very refreshing oil, enabling one to feel awake and cheerful, while relaxed. Soothing to the nervous and digestive system, when added to a massage blend, it will draw the stiffness out of sore, tense muscles. It is a good cleanser of the blood that will detoxify and rejuvenate the skin, returning to it the quality of youth.
Caution: Orange essential oil may cause photosensitivity in sunlight and may irritate sensitive skins.

PATCHOULI
(Pogostemon patchouli)

Erotic

Patchouli has a deep, musky, and lingering aroma that is associated both with earthy sensuality and spiritual elevation. It has always enjoyed a reputation of being a sexually provocative perfume – growing in popularity during the Sixties and becoming the aroma of choice during the hippie era of "free love." Many patchouli incense sticks were burned in the bedrooms of young people keen to explore the new world of sexual freedom.

Patchouli gives off a scent that is either loved or hated. An ingredient in love potions and magic charms throughout the ages, it is reputed to be an aphrodisiac of magical powers. The sensual musky aroma that it emits decreases inhibition, allowing people to succumb to the earthy pleasures of the body's innate sexuality. While encouraging desire, this essential oil will enable a person to communicate more clearly about their physical and emotional needs. It can uplift and nourish the spirit and has been combined

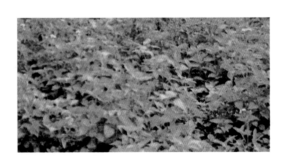

with both sandalwood and frankincense to aid meditation and contemplation. Patchouli originated in Malaysia and India. Now it is also grown in the West Indies, China, Indonesia, and Paraguay.

The essence has been widely used in perfumery as a fixative, and Indian women include patchouli in a variety of cosmetics. Patchouli is a nurturing oil when someone is in a state of anxiety and depression. It can be either stimulating or sedative, depending on the degree of its dosage.

There are no known precautions.

ROSE ABSOLUTE
(*Rosa centifolia/damascena/gallica*)

Erotic

The beautiful rose is the symbol of Venus, the Goddess of Love. No

higher honor could be given to this lovely flower, whose fragrance has

long been admired for its aphrodisiac and sexual healing properties.

It is a perfume that is emotionally uplifting; that has the capacity to

ease the sadness of lost love while soothing away painful feelings.

Rose has a natural affinity with the heart, opening it up

to tender feelings as surely as its petals expand to

embrace the warmth of the sun.

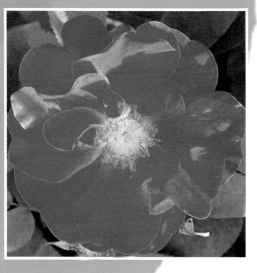

Throughout history, rose has been noted as the

flower of seduction. Legend has it that the wise Queen

Cleopatra first made love with Mark Anthony on a car-

pet buried one inch deep in rose petals. In ancient

Rome and Egypt, rose petals were scattered at wed-

dings to guarantee happiness. The women of the court

of Queen Elizabeth I of England sewed sachets of rose

petals into their skirts to charm gallant courtiers. Even the Victorians

gave red roses to proclaim their passion, a romantic tradition that

still exists to this day.

The essential oil is obtained from rose petals by enfleurage –

the process of exposing odorless oils to the scent of fresh flowers.

The flowers are picked just after the early morning dew when their

therapeutic and fragrant properties are at their peak. As this process

yields so little oil, it is expensive. Rose oil has a special connection

with the female reproductive system and helps to ease frigidity.

Caution: Use of rose absolute is best avoided during pregnancy.

S A N D A L W O O D
(Santalum Album)

Erotic

Sandalwood's sweet and woody perfume instills the mysteries of the East wherever its aroma fills the air. It is another essential oil that encompasses and enhances both the spiritual and physical well-being of men and women.

Burned as a temple incense in worship to the gods, in India sandalwood paste has been used in spiritual and ritualistic sexual practices. Tantric disciples smeared it onto their bodies while celebrating the divinity of sexual ecstasy. The Hindu love scripture, the *Kama Sutra*, which graphically details the positions of lovemaking, also refers to the use of ointments and woods – almost certainly derived from sandalwood.

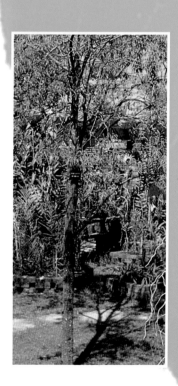

Sandalwood's essence encourages an emotional openness within a relationship, while enhancing physical sensuality. Guiding partners away from the distractions of the mind back to the earthy sensual joy of their bodies, it is a good aphrodisiac. Sandalwood also helps to break old habits of thought and behavior, creating a new and spontaneous interaction between lovers, leading them out of the rut of stuck sexual patterns.

In both India and Egypt, sandalwood was added to cosmetics to preserve the beauty and youth of women. A powerful aid to meditation, sandalwood can help release someone from the grip of anxiety, worry, and guilt, bringing them back to a feeling of inner peace. In skincare it is particularly beneficial in the relief of irritated skin and has excellent properties for dry and mature skin.

There are no known precautions.

YLANG YLANG
(Cananga odorata)

Erotic

The sweet, heady fragrance of ylang ylang acts as a powerful aphrodisiac, increasing libido and enhancing attraction between lovers. Its sensual and seductive reputation has caused it to become a honeymoon symbol in Indonesia, where ylang ylang flowers are scattered over the bed sheets of newlyweds for the benefit of both bride and groom. In the South Sea Islands, the flowers are worn in the hair and woven into necklaces on the wedding day.

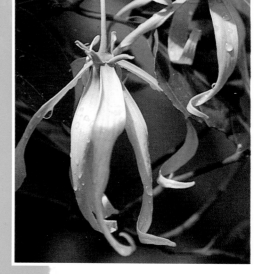

The essential oil of this rich, heady, and exotic flower works its magic on the heart and nervous system, which is why it has become relevant to love and libido. In lovemaking, it soothes the over-anxious and over-excited, while boosting low energy. Its healing properties are believed to help both impotence and frigidity. Ylang ylang resonates on the heart, opening the emotions and the inner self.

Emotionally this essential oil can calm feelings of anger, shock, panic, and fear, making it a true friend in times of difficulty, change, and upheaval. It also soothes feelings of jealousy, frustration and, irritation. Thus used in a lover's recipe, ylang ylang has the effect of opening the mind and spirit to a more sensual and erotic experience during lovemaking.

Ylang ylang's essence is beneficial to both oily and dry skin, and can be used as a toner to firm the breasts.

Caution: Some people find that a high dilution of the rich sweet fragrance can give them a headache or cause nausea.

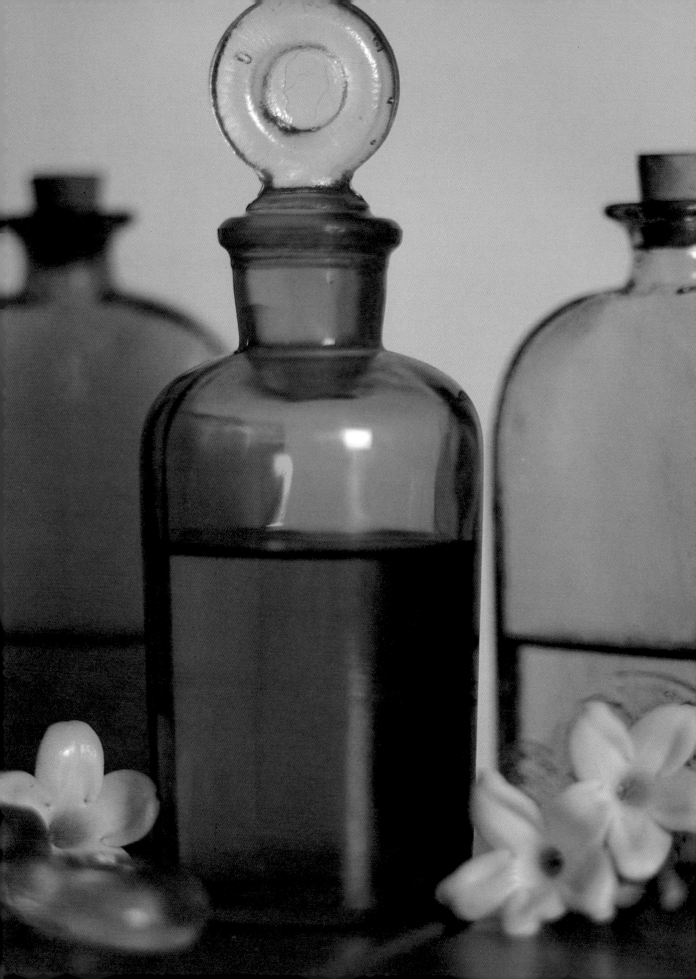

THE BASE OILS OF AROMATHERAPY

The base oil recipes mentioned throughout this book refer to the vegetable oils into which the essential oils are blended. By adding the aromatic essences to one or a combination of recommended base oils, the benefits of the essential oils are spread out over a larger area of the body and can penetrate a wider surface of skin. Essential oils are very potent and should never be applied directly to the skin. By adding the drops to a base oil mixture, their potency can be suitably diluted so as not to contact the skin directly.

Base oils can be used with or without the addition of essential oils to facilitate a massage. They provide the necessary lubrication on the skin to make sure that massage strokes can be performed in a sensual and flowing manner. This is particularly important to allow the hands to sculpt and mold to the body contours, while enhancing the soothing and nourishing aspect of a loving and tender touch.

The base oils recommended in this book also provide nutrition for the skin as they contain the essential fatty acids and vitamins required to maintain the health of the skin. There are differences in the thickness and texture between the oils, and some are more appropriate for certain skin types than others. The seven base oils mentioned in the essential oil recipes in this book are listed below, together with their specific properties and uses.

The base oils, otherwise known as carrier oils, can be obtained from health-food stores and should be non-refined cold-pressed oils, rather than heat-treated oils. Remember to store them in the refrigerator once the bottle has been opened.

Almond Oil: This oil has a somewhat sticky texture, but it can be used alone, or added to a lighter vegetable oil such as grapeseed or sunflower to enrich it. Almond oil contains a variety of vitamins and minerals, most notably Vitamin D. Suitable for all skin types.

Avocado Oil: A nutrient-rich base oil with a high content of vitamins, protein, lecithin, and essential fatty acids. It has a fairly thick texture and is better used when added to a lighter vegetable oil blend. Especially suitable for mature, wrinkled, dry, and itchy skin.

Grapeseed Oil: A popular choice for a massage blend because it has a light texture and can be easily absorbed by the skin, suiting all skin types. Non-odoriferous, this oil is greatly enhanced by the addition of more nutritious oils, such as almond.

Jojoba Oil: An oil rich in Vitamin E, which can be used alone or mixed with other base oils. Suitable for all skin types.

Olive Oil: A nutrient-rich oil, containing Vitamin E that is excellent for treating sore, dry, or chapped skin. It is not a popular choice of oil for aromatherapy massage owing to its sticky, thick texture, and its strong odor. Occasional use as a treatment for dry skin or as a hand treatment, however, will be beneficial.

Sunflower Oil: This oil is a popular choice for massage. Its light, non-sticky texture means that it can be used alone or blended with richer oils.

Wheat Germ Oil: An antioxidant oil; adding a small proportion of it to a basic mix will retain the freshness of the blend. It is particularly beneficial to dry and mature skin as it is rich in Vitamin E.

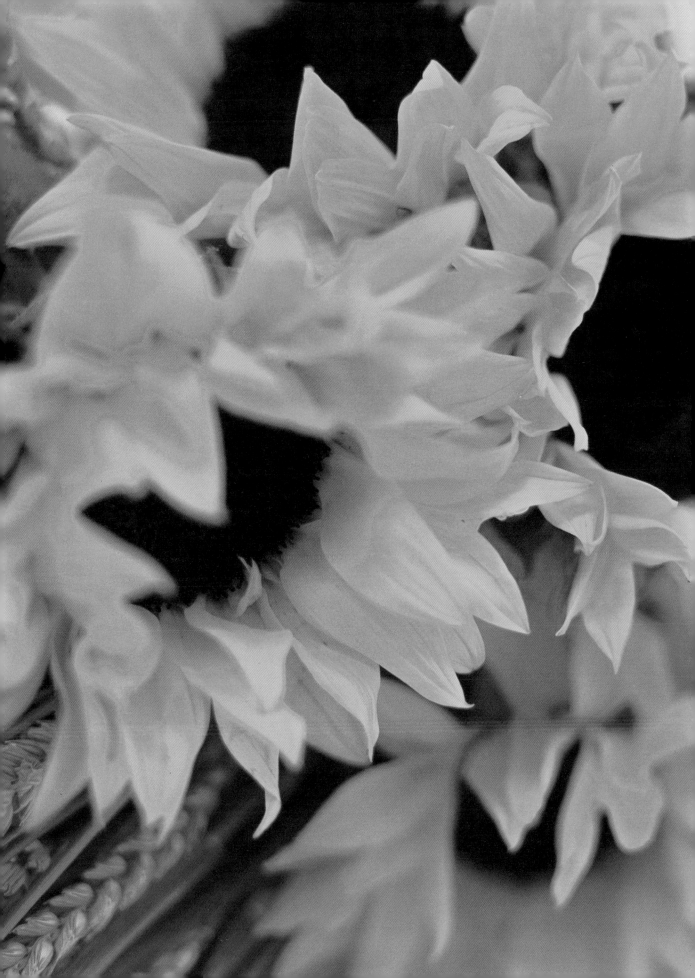

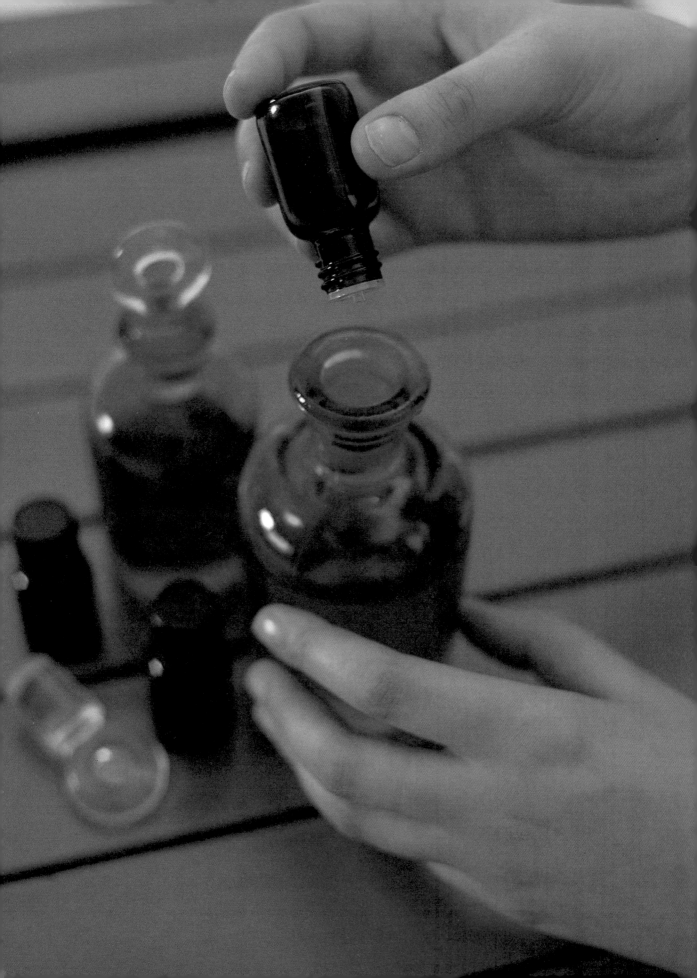

BLENDING AND STORING

Essential oils are both volatile and delicate, and their chemical make-up will change if exposed to sun or air, detrimentally affecting their therapeutic value. Store bottles of essential oils in dark glass containers away from sunlight and, if possible, in a cool place. Always replace the cap on the bottle directly after use. Once the essential oils are added to a pure vegetable oil base, the efficacy of the blend will last for several months if stored in a glass bottle with its cap securely placed, or for one day if it has been mixed in a glass or ceramic bowl. Remember, that essential oils should not be kept in plastic containers.

Patch Tests: A patch test before use is recommended to be sure that a particular essential oil is suitable to a sensitive or allergy-prone skin. Put one drop of the essential oil on a pad of cotton wool and gently stroke over a small area of skin on the inside of the arm. Do not wash this area for 24 hours. If there is any itchiness, redness, or any other type of allergic reaction, do not use this essential oil.

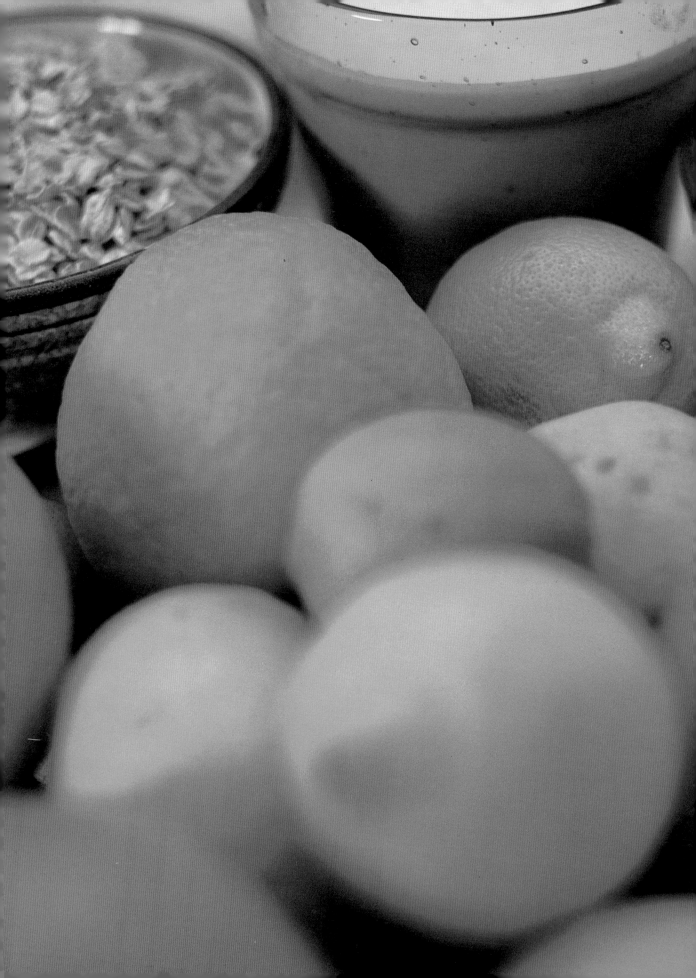

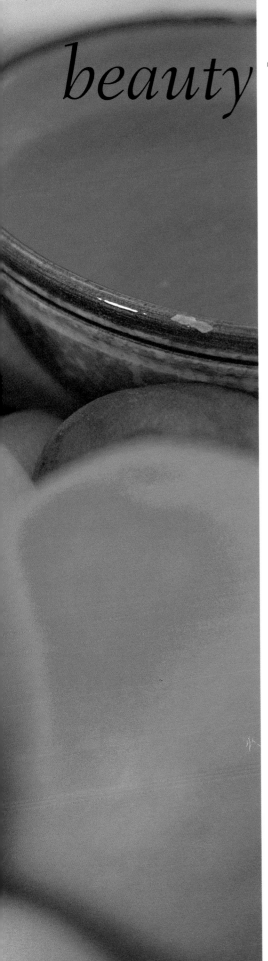

beauty treatments

Since ancient times, perfumes and ingredients extracted from plant essences have been mixed with nutrient-rich oils, such as olive and almond, and animal fat to be rubbed into the body for beauty, seduction, and love. Skin-care products were used in ancient Egypt, and when Tutankhamun's tomb was excavated, archaeologists discovered a 3000-year-old skin cream consisting of animal fat and perfumed resin.

When it comes to skin and body care, nature has a healing, soothing, cleansing, and replenishing potency with which few synthetic cosmetics can compare. These natural ingredients are pure, alive and vital, rich in vitamins, minerals and enzymes that nurture new cells, extract impurities and maintain the skin's natural pH balance. They can also help to ward off the damaging environmental effects caused to the skin by the sun's rays, chemicals, and pollution. After a period in which synthetic chemicals have dominated the cosmetic and beauty industry, many people are again preferring to choose products containing natural ingredients.

Many of nature's healing agents are readily available in your kitchen. Nuts, fruits, vegetables, oils, fats, herbs, live yogurt, oatmeal, and honey are just some of the products that can form the base of skincare preparations. Add to those a few useful utensils for blending, and with the right essential oil recipes to suit your skin type, you can create a health and beauty farm within your own home.

Many of the aphrodisiac essential oils described in this book are also beneficial to skin care. Some others, not mentioned in the Chapter 1, are particularly renowned for their skin healing properties, so they have been included in the list below, which matches essential oils most appropriate to certain skin types or conditions:

Normal Skin: Frankincense, Geranium, Jasmine, Lavender, Palmarosa, Patchouli, Chamomile, Rose, Sandalwood.

Oily Skin: Bergamot, Cedarwood, Cypress, Frankincense, Geranium, Grapefruit, Juniper, Lime, Ylang Ylang.

Dry Skin: Carrot, Chamomile, Geranium, Jasmine, Lavender, Neroli, Palmarosa, Rose, Sandalwood.

Combination Skin: Geranium, Lavender, Jasmine, Palmarosa, Rose.

Mature Skin: Carrot, Cypress, Frankincense, Geranium, Lavender, Neroli, Palmarosa, Rose, Rosewood.

Acned Skin: Bergamot, Cedarwood, Juniper, Lavender, Patchouli, Tea Tree.

Chapped/Cracked Skin: Benzoin, Carrot, Geranium, Lavender, Patchouli.

Sensitive Skin: Chamomile, Lavender, Neroli, Rose.

If using essential oils in skincare regularly, use them at a low dilution. The correct dilution is 1 drop to 1tsp or 2 drops of essential oil to every 2tsp of base oil or unperfumed lotion used.

RECIPES FOR SKIN CLEANSERS

RECIPE 1
Floral Water for Skin without Make-up

To 5tsp of distilled water add 5 drops of one of the following essential oils:
Rose, Chamomile, Neroli, Lavender
Close bottle firmly and always shake well before use to mix the oil and water.

FACE CLEANSING

A balanced lifestyle with adequate sleep, healthy diet, and plenty of exercise is the best tonic for the skin. A high nutritional intake of fresh fruits and vegetables, plus fiber and lots of pure water, will nourish and cleanse your internal organs and have a positive and glowing effect on the skin. Daily care of the skin is also important to cleanse, replenish, and protect it from damaging environmental factors that can cause it to age prematurely. The essential oil preparations recommended on these pages, combined with other natural ingredients, are particularly suitable because they are readily absorbed into the skin. They promote healthy cell generation, and their action on sebum production (oily secretion from sebaceous glands in the skin) means that their use can benefit all skin types.

Cleanse your skin twice a day, once in the morning to remove dead cells and toxins and once at night to lift away make-up, dirt, and other impurities. Floral water, obtained from drugstores and health-food stores or made at home (see Recipe 1), is a good skin cleanser when rubbed over the face with a cotton ball.

RECIPE 2
Cleanser for Skin with Make-up

To 1tbs unperfumed cleansing cream or lotion add:

For oily skin:
1 drop Juniper

For dry skin:
1 drop Palmarosa

For normal skin:
1 drop Lavender

For mature skin:
1 drop of either Rose, Chamomile, or Carrot

Add and mix 1 drop of essential oil to every 2tsp of unperfumed lotion directly into its container or transfer 2tsp to a smaller jar. Stir well with a cotton swab and seal firmly between use.

RECIPES FOR STEAMING

RECIPE 1

Normal to Dry Skin

Sandalwood, Chamomile

To bowl of

steaming water add:

2 drops Sandalwood

3 drops Chamomile

RECIPE 2

Normal to Oily Skin

Juniper, Geranium

To bowl of

steaming water add:

2 drops Juniper,

3 drops Geranium

RECIPES FOR FACE MASKS

RECIPE 1

Normal to Dry Skin

To a mashed banana add:

2tbs oatmeal.

Rosewater to make a paste.

Spread mask on face. Leave

for 10-20 minutes.

Face steaming with an essential oil infusion is another excellent method of cleansing the skin and removing toxins. It stimulates the blood circulation, softening and loosening excess sebum that can clog the pores. You can steam your face once a week, but people with sensitive skins or dilated capillaries should seek professional beauty therapy advice before steaming.

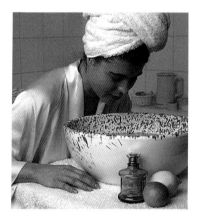

THE AROMATIC INFUSION WILL SOFTLY CLEANSE YOUR SKIN

Fill a bowl with steaming boiled water and add up to 5 drops of your selected essential oils (see Recipes). Being very careful not to tip the bowl, put a towel over your head to trap the steam. Close your eyes and enjoy the relaxing sensation of warm steam on your face for between 3 to 5 minutes. After steaming, splash your face with cold water and pat dry with a towel. Then apply a moisturizer (see overleaf).

Concocting your own face mask from your kitchen ingredients is a fun and inexpensive beauty preparation. Face masks can be applied once a week to exfoliate – draw out impurities and act as an astringent. Look to your kitchen stock for the base of your mask. Avocado is rich in minerals and vitamins, and is nourishing to dry or mature skin. Banana moisturizes and softens, especially if your skin has been exposed to the sun. Live yogurt suits combination

and oily skins, cleansing and tightening it. Honey is soothing and
healing, and oatmeal, when crushed in a blender, is a gentle exfo-
liant suitable for all skin types, but particularly effective if skin is dry,
allergic, or chapped. Mineral-rich clays such as kaolin or Fuller's
earth, readily available from most pharmacies, are completely natural
cleansing agents, drawing toxins out from deep within the skin.

Check the face mask recipes to choose a blend that suits you
best, and mix the ingredients into a glass or ceramic bowl, adding
the appropriate drops of flower water or essential oils. Use a
wooden spoon to stir into a firm paste. Spread the mask all over
your face except for the delicate skin below your eyes. Leave on for
ten to twenty minutes, depending on your choice of recipe, while
you relax or continue your tasks – then wash off and moisturize.

RECIPE 2
Normal to Oily Skin
Geranium, Lemon
To ¹/2 cup blend of live
yogurt, enough crushed oats
to make a thick paste, and
1tsp of warmed honey add:
1 drop Geranium
1 drop Lemon
Leave mask on face for
up to 10-20 minutes

RECIPE 3
Mature Skin or Dry Skin
Rose, Chamomile, or Carrot
To thick paste of pulped half
of avocado, 2tbs of jojoba oil,
1 capsule Evening Primrose
oil and 2tbs of
heavy cream add:
1 drop Rose
1 drop Chamomile or Carrot
Leave on for up to
15 minutes

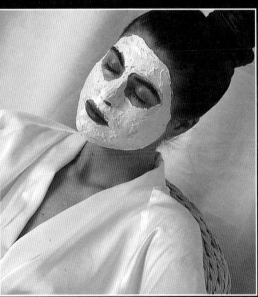

**CLOSE YOUR EYES AND
RELAX AS THE MASK DRIES
ON YOUR SKIN**

MOISTURIZING
AND MASSAGING
THE FACE

To get the maximum benefit from moisturizing and massaging your face, you will need to make this part of your daily skincare routine. Add your aromatic or soothing essential oils to a base oil mix consisting of pure vegetable or nut oils rather than petroleum-based ones, as the former are vitamin-rich and more readily absorbed into the deeper layers of the skin. Combine 2tsp of jojoba oil with 2tsp of sweet almond oil for a base mix, or for a really moisturizing massage on drier or more mature skin, replace the sweet almond with

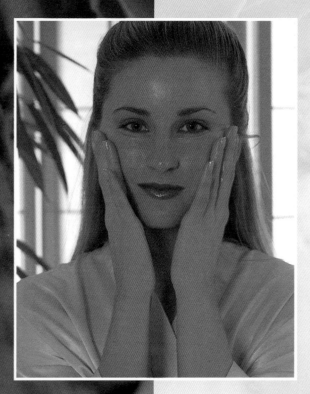

avocado oil. By choosing the appropriate recipe for your skin type, you can soothe dry or chapped areas, balance sebum production, and make your complexion feel fresh, silky, and alive. When applying moisturizer to the face, remember to include your neck. Early skincare and massage of the neck can help to reduce a double chin and reduce signs of aging such as lines and wrinkles.

A self massage on the face and neck in the morning will refresh you for the day ahead and, at night, will ease away tension and the effects of stress. The rhythmic stroking of your fingertips over your features will enliven your skin, drawing the blood circulation close to its surface to nourish tissues and cells. If you use sensual aromatic essences in your moisturizing blend, their fragrance will linger with you all day.

With clean hands, smooth the moisturizing oil all over your face and neck. If choosing Recipe 1 or 2, use your middle fingers to dab the oil under your eyes. Allow it to soak in without massaging so you do not disturb the delicate tissues. Smooth the oil over your face with soft and flowing movements from your palms and fingers. Relax your hands so they are able to trace and sculpt the contours of your face. The flowing and rhythmic motion of your hands soon begin to warm the muscles and tissues that lay beneath them.

Now add strokes to stimulate the skin and ease away tension. Focus first on your brow and temples. Circulate your fingertips over the forehead, moving both hands out from the center to the sides of your head. Stroke your fingers simultaneously around both temples to clear and ease your mind. Press and squeeze along the rims of both ears with your thumbs and index finger, and then stroke behind the ears. Sweep both hands in a soft, counter-clockwise motion over your cheeks, then work deeper with fingertip circles over the cheeks and jaw. Now tone the skin and stimulate its circulation by tapping the fingertips of both hands rhythmically all over the face, starting on the forehead and then vibrating them over the temples, cheekbones, cheeks, jaw, and chin. Finally, rhythmically tap below your chin and jaw with the back of one hand. Wipe the excess oil from your hands and continue tapping all over your scalp for a truly revitalizing finish.

RECIPES FOR THE FACE

RECIPE 1

Truly Pampering

Rose, Jasmine

To 4tsp base oil mix of jojoba and sweet almond or avocado base oil mix add:

3 drops Rose

1 drop Jasmine

RECIPE 2

Deeply Moisturizing

Sandalwood, Carrot, Lavender

To above-mentioned base oil mix add:

1 drop Sandalwood

1 drop Carrot

2 drops Lavender

HAND CARE

RECIPES FOR HAND CARE

RECIPE 1

Moisturizing

Patchouli, Geranium, Lavender

To 1tbs of
unperfumed hand lotion or
1tbs of olive oil add:
1 drop Patchouli
2 drops Geranium
1 drop Lavender

RECIPE 2

To Soften and Perfume

Carrot, Rose, Neroli

To each 1tbs of
unperfumed hand cream
or lotion add:
1 drop Carrot
1 drop Rose
1 drop Neroli

Our hands express our creativity. We use them constantly in every aspect of our daily lives. The hands contain many thousands of sensory nerve receptors that relay all kinds of sensations back to our brain. Through our arms and hands, we reach out to the world to touch people, objects, and the ones we love. Keeping our hands supple and dextrous is important to all of our functions. So, too, is their appearance, for beautifully cared-for hands say much about a person's sense of self-worth. Even when manual work causes stains or wear and tear on the hands, careful precautions and grooming with creams, oil, and aromatic essences can restore them to peak condition. If you put your hands in hot water to do the household chores, work in the yard, or use industrial oils and chemicals, always protect your hands by wearing gloves.

The recipes for hand care on this page will keep them fragrant and smooth. Regular hand massage and nail care, using essential essences mixed with pure oils or unperfumed creams, will mean they stay in tip-top condition.

If your hands become chapped or cracked, through cold weather or over-use, soothe them with the luxuriant essences of patchouli, geranium, and lavender (Recipe 1), which are not only very sensual oils, but contain skin healing properties, too. Add them to an unperfumed hand cream, or for special care mix with nutrient-rich olive oil. This oil is generally too sticky for applying to the body, but its excellent properties will work wonders on sore, dry hands. Massage the olive oil blend into your hands and leave to soak into the skin for fifteen minutes, then wipe away excess oil with a soft cloth or towel.

To soften and perfume your hands, or to leave your lingering aroma with someone special with whom you have shaken or held hands, try Recipe 2, which combines carrot oil with the essences of rose and neroli. The combination of carrot and rose essences not only soothe the skin, but blend together to make an enticing odor.

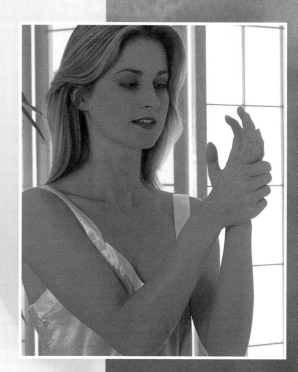

Take care of your nails and you will be rewarded with great-looking hands. Your nutritional intake will have the biggest impact on their health. To condition your nails, rub them with the blend of oils listed in Recipe 3, allowing it to soak in for a couple of hours before washing your hands or polishing your nails.

REGULARLY MASSAGE EACH PART OF YOUR HANDS

Massage your hands daily when you apply your aromatic cream or oil, even if only for five minutes on each hand. Stroke over the top and palm of one hand with circular motions from the other hand. Then stroke your thumb with a stronger pressure over both sides to revitalize the circulation, relax muscles and tendons, and to stimulate the nerve endings. Press and squeeze the hand all over between your fingers and heel. Then wiggle and flex wrist and finger joints to make them supple. Use your thumb and index finger to stretch firmly along each digit from its base to tip.

RECIPE 3

Conditioning Nails

Lemon, Palmarosa

To 1tsp avocado oil

mixed with 1tsp of

jojoba oil add:

1 drop lemon oil

1 drop Palmarosa

FOOT CARE

The feet are generally the most neglected part of the body in terms of beauty care, probably because they are usually hidden from view. Yet beautiful, soft, and well-groomed feet can be an exquisite turn-on, especially when rubbed seductively against the skin of a lover. Taking good care of your feet will be rewarding in many ways. First, by pampering and applying lotions, creams, or oils, blended with especially selected essences (see Recipe 1), you can relax and soften the feet, helping to prevent tough, dry areas of skin from building up.

An essential oil known as tea-tree has long been used by the aboriginal peoples of Australia for its antiseptic properties and works well to protect the feet from fungal infections. Adding two drops of tea-tree and three of lavender to a warm foot bath and soaking your feet in it for ten minutes will be both relaxing to you and a real treat for your feet.

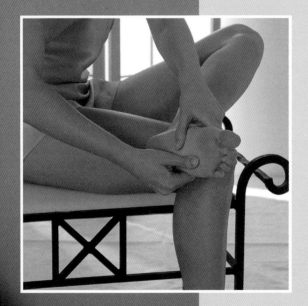

Feet, cooped up in socks and shoes, tend to get hot, sweaty, and tired by the end of the day. Bathe and then massage your feet with the ingredients in Recipe 2 to ease the strain and weariness from them. The soles are particularly porous and able to absorb the benefits of the essential oils. Pressing, rubbing, and stroking your feet in a self-massage will revitalize your whole system, removing tension from the muscles and tendons while bringing greater relaxation to the whole body posture as stress dissolves away.

Sit comfortably to apply the massage, laying the calf of one leg over the thigh of the other to gain good access to both sides of your foot. Cradle the foot between both hands for a few moments to give it warmth and then briskly rub both hands back and forth to create a heat-producing friction. Spread it over the foot with soothing sweeps, gliding your hands smoothly over the foot's shapely contours. If you want to apply deeper pressure, use the oil sparingly so the foot does not become too slippery.

Stroke all around your foot, ankle joint, and heel with your palms, fingers, thumbs, and heels. Squeeze and press the foot to gently manipulate its many bones, stretching and releasing tension from tendons and muscles. If you are tired and in need of a boost of energy, focus your strokes on the sole of your foot. Thumb pressure will activate the nerve endings, boost your circulation, and can, according to some therapists, stimulate energy pathways to have a beneficial effect on all aspects of body and mind. Using both thumbs, work them over the sole of the foot, with strong alternating circular motions. Or you can press one thumb, spot by spot, all over its surface. Use fingers and thumb to gently rotate the joints in each toe and then wiggle them up and down. Make little corkscrew motions with your little finger on the delicate skin between each toe. Then press and squeeze along each toe, before giving each a stretch by gripping firmly between thumb and finger and pulling steadily up to its tip. For a relaxing finish, cradle the foot in both hands before repeating the strokes on the other foot.

RECIPES FOR FOOT CARE

RECIPE 1

To Soften and Relax

Palmarosa, Bergamot, Benzoin

To base oil mix of

2tsp grapeseed and

1tsp sweet

almond oil add:

1 drop Palmarosa

1 drop Bergamot

1 drop Benzoin

RECIPE 2

Revitalizing

Peppermint, Tea-Tree, Orange

To base oil mix mentioned

above add:

1 drop Peppermint

1 drop Tea-Tree

2 drops Orange

BREAST
AND CHEST CARE

RECIPES FOR BREAST AND CHEST CARE

RECIPE 1
Breast Care for
Women
Rose, Geranium
To base oil mix of 1tsp
grapeseed and 2tsp sweet
almond add:
2 drops Rose
1 drop Geranium

RECIPE 2
Chest Care for Men
Sandalwood, Lavender
To base oil mix of above
mentioned ingredients add:
2 drops Sandalwood
1 drop Lavender

For women, the breasts are a very intimate and feminine part of the body and deserve to receive the best of attention. The chest area, however, is an erogenous zone for both sexes and plays an erotic part in touching and lovemaking. Essential oils will keep this area toned, as well as soft and fragranced with the odors of love.

Many women have concerns about their breast shape and size. Although the shape and size of an individual's breasts are largely determined by genes, massage and essential oils can enhance their tone and feel. The breasts are glands and, unlike muscles, cannot be enlarged or shaped by exercise, although improved posture and working out can lift the pectoral muscles to give them better definition. Loving and accepting your breasts the way they are is an important part of becoming a woman. Tending to them with aromatic massage can help the process of acceptance, while also keeping them soft and reducing the risk of stretch marks.

Recipe 1 on these pages is especially for women, because it uses the deeply feminine essence of rose, flower of love and healer of the heart. It is a particularly appropriate essential oil for this part of your body, as well as being a tonic for the circulatory, digestive, and nervous systems. Combined with the rich, floral aroma of geranium, it makes an excellent recipe for toning and breast skin care. Geranium helps to balance the hormonal functions of the body and can ease premenstrual tension and painful breasts. It is acceptable to all skin types and is frequently used to soften and help skin when pores have become clogged and congested.

Recipe 2 has been selected for men to combine with massage to tone muscles and soften skin on the chest. Both sandalwood and lavender are soothing to skin. The woody aroma of sandalwood is very acceptable to men as a perfume. The chest is an area where your lover may want to rest her head, to nuzzle into you, and to feel secure. If your chest feels soft and smooth and fragrant with the evocative and sensual smell of sandalwood, it will provide her with a luxurious pillow.

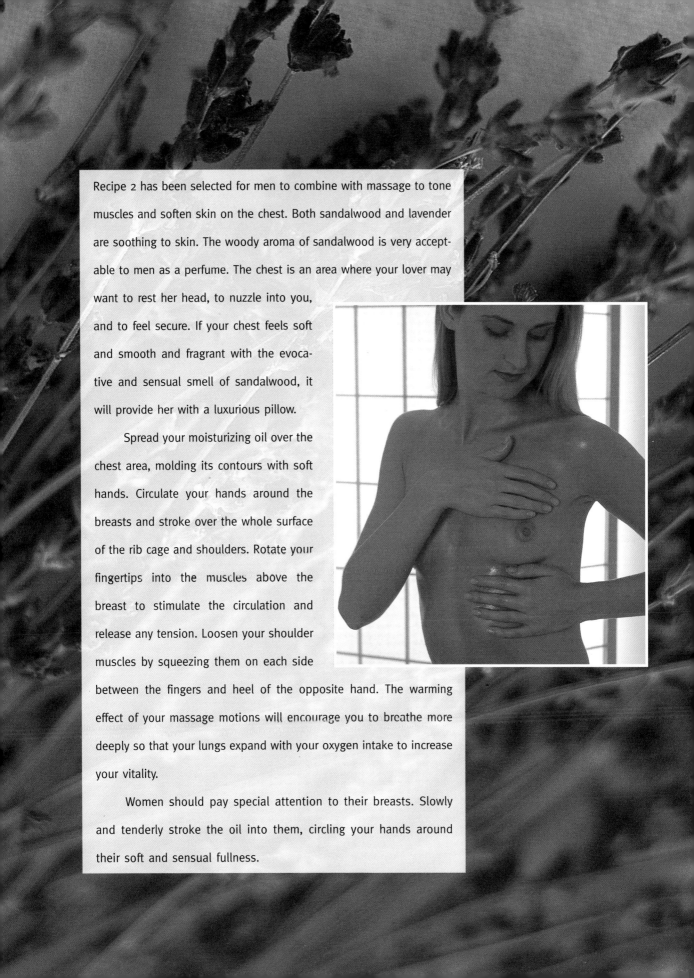

Spread your moisturizing oil over the chest area, molding its contours with soft hands. Circulate your hands around the breasts and stroke over the whole surface of the rib cage and shoulders. Rotate your fingertips into the muscles above the breast to stimulate the circulation and release any tension. Loosen your shoulder muscles by squeezing them on each side between the fingers and heel of the opposite hand. The warming effect of your massage motions will encourage you to breathe more deeply so that your lungs expand with your oxygen intake to increase your vitality.

Women should pay special attention to their breasts. Slowly and tenderly stroke the oil into them, circling your hands around their soft and sensual fullness.

BEAUTIFYING
THE THIGHS

The thighs, being so close to the very intimate sexual areas, are an erogenous zone in the body. For both men and women, tender touches, kisses, and strokes on the thighs can lead to a heightening of sexual arousal. Good tone and strength in the thigh muscles helps to enhance lovemaking by supporting the pelvic movements. Massage and moisturizing the thighs with a blend of essential oils, renowned not only for their aphrodisiac aromas, but for their skin care properties, will certainly increase their sensuality. In Recipe 1, the suggested oil blend includes the exotic and musky perfume of patchouli mixed with the haunting, bittersweet fragrance of neroli – the orange blossom oil. Both these evocative oils have long been used for their magical and sexually inviting qualities. Patchouli is said to be a helpful essence for many skin complaints, as well as having skin regenerating properties. Neroli has been used cosmetically by many an alluring woman throughout history – Cleopatra was reputed to be one of its admirers. It is good for dry, sensitive, and mature skin, increasing its elasticity and helping to prevent stretch marks.

To bring softness to your skin and sensuality to your thighs, massage this wonderful preparation into them on a regular basis. Spread the oil evenly over the thighs and buttocks, taking particular care to be gentle with the skin along your inner thighs.

STROKE THE OIL SMOOTHLY

ONTO YOUR THIGHS

Ideally, thighs should be firm in tone and silky to touch. Many women, however, suffer from cellulite in these areas, a condition which causes fleshy parts of the body to have a bumpy orange-peel look. Cellulite results from a sluggish lymphatic circulation that fails to eliminate excess fluids and toxins accumulated in fat cells. The condition is helped by regular aromatic massage, but will only be effective in combination with a change to a healthy diet and regular exercise. If you have cellulite, massage daily with the oils in Recipe 2 that have been selected for their stimulating, diuretic, tonic, and purifying properties.

Start a massage to help break down the cellulite by placing the foot on a chair to raise your knee. This helps the lymph system carry dispersing toxins to the lymph glands in the groin. Working on one leg at a time, spread the oil over the thigh and warm up the muscles with circular strokes. Then use pummeling strokes to break down fatty deposits. Make loose fists and with their sides, strike briskly over the thigh, bouncing one hand after the other off the skin in rapid succession. Sweep your hands over the thigh, moving the strokes toward the groin.

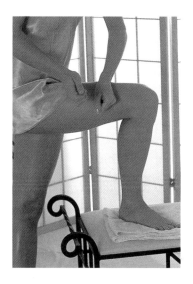

PUMMEL BRISKLY TO

DISPERSE TOXINS

RECIPES FOR BEAUTIFYING THE THIGHS

RECIPE 1

Sensuality

Patchouli, Neroli

To 2tsp base oil mix of 1tsp each of jojoba and grapeseed oil add:

1 drop Patchouli

3 drops Neroli

RECIPE 2

Cellulite Massage

Rosemary, Geranium, Lemon, Juniper

To base oil mix of 2tbs sweet almond and 1tsp wheatgerm add:

4 drops Rosemary

4 drops Geranium

4 drops Lemon

4 drops Juniper

HAIR CARE

RECIPES FOR HAIR CARE

RECIPE 1

Conditioner
for Dry/Out-of-
Condition Hair

Geranium, Lavender

To base oil mix of 2tsp

sweet almond add:

2 drops Geranium

1 drop Lavender

RECIPE 2

Conditioner for
Greasy Hair

Bergamot, Lavender

To base oil mix mentioned

in Recipe 1 add:

2 drops Bergamot

1 drop Lavender

Just like your skin and nails, the condition of your hair is greatly affected by your overall state of well-being. A healthy lifestyle, including a balanced diet with plenty of protein and amino acids, plus vitamins, and minerals, will add luster and shine to a head of hair.

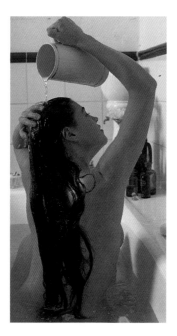

RINSE AND CONDITION YOUR HAIR

Many essential oils will enhance the condition of your hair, whether it is normal, dry, or greasy. You can combine them with nutrient-rich sweet almond oil to make a conditioner and tonic for your hair and scalp. Massaging the scalp is a very important part of caring for your hair. It will stimulate the blood circulation to the hair follicles and release the tightness of the scalp muscles that is often a common but unrecognized tension resulting from stress. Try giving your head a massage every morning, and you will be amazed by its revitalizing effects. It need take only a few minutes, but it will refresh and awaken you for the new day.

What you must aim to do is to ease and move the scalp muscles that lie over the skull. Work your fingertips thoroughly over your scalp, from where the ridge of the skull meets the neck, to the crown of your head. Make circular shampooing movements to cover every inch of the scalp. Then vibrate your fingers back and forth on the scalp to create a heat-producing friction. Bend over for a few seconds to let the blood supply move to your head while you continue to stimulate your scalp with your fingers.

A conditioning combination of eucalyptus and rosemary is excellent for treating dandruff (see Recipe 3) as it will warm and tone the scalp and boost the circulation. For hair loss, clary sage combined with rosemary will also provide a stimulating tonic for the head and hair, with the bonus of clearing and refreshing the mind.

To deep-condition the hair, add the essential oils suggested in the recipes to the base of sweet almond oil and massage it into the scalp and hair for five minutes. Then wrap your hair in a warm towel for twenty minutes. If you soak in a warm bath for this time, the added heat from the steam will increase the absorption of the oils. Wash your hair thoroughly afterward and then condition it as usual.

USE YOUR FINGERTIPS TO DISTRIBUTE CONDITIONER

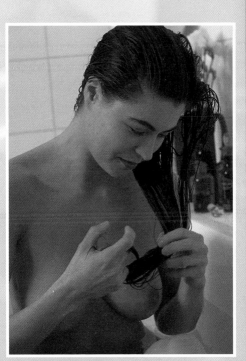

RECIPE 3
Conditioner for
Dandruff
Eucalyptus, Rosemary
To base oil mentioned in
Recipe 1 add:
2 drops Eucalyptus
1 drop Rosemary

RECIPE 4
Conditioner for
Hair Loss
Clary Sage, Rosemary
To base oil mentioned in
Recipe 1 add:
1 drop Clary Sage
2 drops Rosemary

RECIPES FOR SENSUAL BATHING

RECIPE 1

Relaxing

Patchouli, Sandalwood,

Lavender

To a tub of bathwater add:

2 drops Patchouli

3 drops Sandalwood

3 drops Lavender

RECIPE 2

Sensual and Playful

Frankincense, Orange,

Ylang Ylang

To a tub of bathwater add:

3 drops Frankincense

1 drop Orange

2 drops Ylang Ylang

RECIPE 3

Revitalizing

Rosemary, Lime, Lavender

To a tub of bathwater add:

2 drops Rosemary

2 drops Lime

3 drops Lavender

Bathing, though it may be an everyday event, has many soothing and therapeutic qualities. Soaking in the warmth of the water is cleansing and purifying to the skin, while the heat eases away stress and tension from the body and mind. For many busy people, the period spent bathing is precious time alone away from the demands of their lives, an opportunity to restore an inner sense of peace and quiet.

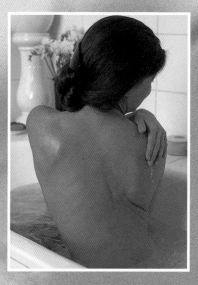

THE COMBINATION OF WARM WATER AND OILS WILL RELAX YOU

Turning your bathing routine into a special occasion will create the opportunity for you to relax and enjoy pampering your body. Turn to Chapter 3, Sensual Ambience, to see how you can turn your bathroom into a welcoming and luxurious temple of sensual delight. When you have selected your oils, place the drops into the bath after the water has stopped running so they do not evaporate too quickly in the steam. Also, be undressed and ready to enter the bath so you can enjoy the full impact of their aroma. Before getting into the water, thoroughly agitate it by hand to disperse and dilute the drops.

If your muscles are sore and aching, then choose Recipe 1 to allow the combination of patchouli, sandalwood, and lavender to soothe and ease away tension, while leaving it perfumed with its sensual and evocative smell. If you have a special date or a party in mind, then luxuriate in the essences of frankincense, orange, and ylang ylang. Frankincense will elevate your spirits and heighten your senses; orange will add cheer and zest, while ylang ylang's sweet exotic smell will induce a feeling of well-being.

**PAMPER YOURSELF
WITH SELF-MASSAGE
AS YOU BATHE**

If you bathe in the morning and need a blend of essential oils to give you a pick-up for the day ahead, choose Recipe 3 for its revitalizing properties. Rosemary will stimulate your circulation; the lime will refresh you, and the lavender, when combined with rosemary, will impart its stimulating qualities, providing a boost to your whole system.

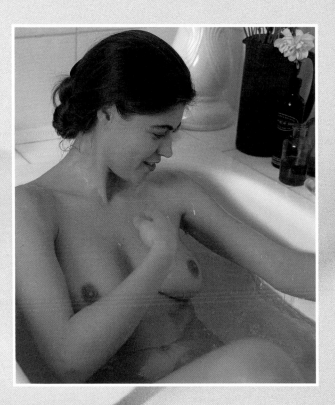

Lie back and enjoy your aromatic bath, letting the oils soothe and soften your skin, while their fragrance lifts your mood. Play with the water, pouring it over your skin and letting it wash away your concerns. Then as your muscles begin to relax, take advantage of your nakedness to apply a few massage strokes to your body. Stroke, squeeze, and press over the areas you can easily reach. Give yourself a face massage. This is also a good opportunity to massage your arms to stimulate their circulation and stroke away their tension.

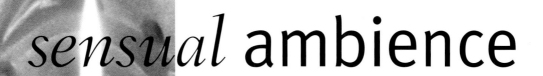

sensual ambience

Creating a sensual ambience for yourself and your partner signifies a respect for the natural beauty of life. The essential oils can be used to invite nature's bounty into your home. Selected carefully, they recreate the richness of the forests, gardens, and meadows and will enhance your feelings of relaxation, romance, and love. When those fragrances are combined with the presence of flowers, candles, and other ambient tools, then many areas of your life can begin to be transformed. In this chapter, you will learn how to use aromatic essences in many different ways, so that any room in your house can be influenced to imbibe the mood of your desire. From practical applications to the romantic, you can choose your own personal scents to improve the quality of your everyday life.

Ideas about how to make your home sensually beautiful cover suggestions on how to use lavender bags, which flowers to choose for each room to suit your moods, and how to select the colors and smells of lovely bowls of potpourri to welcome your guests or brighten your bedroom. Bring romance into your life with fragrant rose-scented bed linen, or transport yourself and your partner to the pleasure gardens of Persia by placing a few drops of the exotic oils into an aromatherapy burner. Use these natural aromas and create a welcoming, warm and evocative home full of atmosphere, harmony and sensuality.

POTPOURRI

Bowls of potpourri displayed throughout a house are another aromatic way of creating a beautiful ambience within your home. The potpourri mixture may be derived from many types of plants – flowers, herbs, spices, nuts, kernels, cones, wood, and leaves. Not only do they infuse a subtle and lingering fragrance into a room, their blend of colors are a pure visual delight. The bowls in which they are laid are also important, for the shape and composition of the receptacle should reflect the nature and essence of the ingredients.

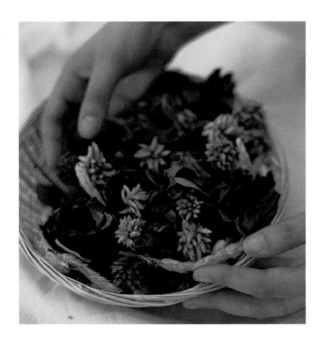

THE COLORS OF POTPOURRI WILL

BRIGHTEN ANY ROOM

Potpourri can come in many shades and hues, though mostly extra color has been added to them by the use of synthetic or vegetable dyes. Color plays an important role as a mood enhancer, so the visual appeal of your potpourri bowl should be in tune with the atmosphere of the room or environment. Additional aroma can be added to the mixture by placing a couple of drops of essential oils onto the dried flowers to complement their character.

A bowl of potpourri placed just inside the front door is a welcome sight for any visitor, and if you add the fragrance of bergamot and lavender essential oil, you can be sure that you have created a happy and inviting perfume for your guests.

Bedroom colors, for the most part, should be soft and restful, such as delicate pinks or gentle shades of blue. In a bowl of potpourri of subtle colors, you could add 1 drop of chamomile and 1 drop of rose. You could also have an exotic blend of red and purple leaves and flowers, which you can lay by your bedside for a romantic night. In this receptacle you can add 1 drop of jasmine and 1 of neroli, to give the potpourri an extra aphrodisiac boost.

Woody pine cones and needles will work in your den, giving the room a character of earthy comfort. Use 2 drops each of cedarwood, geranium, and frankincense, to add a feeling of protection and peace. A wonderful potpourri mix for your bathroom would be an array of dried pods and nuts in the delicate shade of peach, while dried fruit and spices, such as cardamon pods and clove in russets and browns could easily grace your kitchen table. There are so many selections to choose from, that you could use the bowls of potpourri to reflect not only your mood or immediate environments but also the seasons of the year – yellow for spring, green for summer, red for fall, and brown for the winter. A potpourri bowl is very much part of an ambient setting and will look wonderful settled beside your candles and aromatherapy burner.

The art of potpourri is an old one, and many of the wealthy houses in medieval Europe possessed a "still" room, where essential oils were made, and flowers dried. Here the plants of nature were kept and used for their benefits. Herbs and spices were stored in jars, and many flowers were hung to dry from their racks. A room for making potpourri needs to be dark and dry, with good circulation. In a modern house, you could use a closet, shed, or attic.

CANDLES

Every mood-enhancing setting should be bathed in the beautiful glow of candlelight, for the naked flame of a candle is capable of producing a profound change in consciousness, creating an atmosphere that is at once both soporific and inspiring. The image of a burning candle embodies many of our human aspirations – for it has become a symbol of hope and peace, romance and love, devotion and spiritual awareness.

The moment candles are lit and a room becomes swathed in the pure but mellow glow of its light, there is a subtle transformation in mood. Whoever is in that room feels more relaxed and more in harmony with their surroundings. The mind becomes tranquil, and in that stillness, the senses are able to expand and heighten.

That is why candles are burned in churches and temples and places of worship throughout the world. They are lit as offerings and prayers, for the flame of a candle can ascend upward as a perfect pillar of clarity and light. The warm glow of candles will also influence the mood of lovers, for it creates an intimate and romantic ambience in almost any setting. Candlelight is flattering to both the environment and the people within it, smoothing out hard edges and angles, and casting a soft hue onto the skin and a gentle roundness onto the body shape. Its luminosity is perfect when set on a table where lovers will dine, or when placed in a bedroom for a night of passion.

Candles are totally complementary to the use of aromatic essential oils whenever you wish to create a sensual ambience, either for yourself or for you and your partner to share. If you are

bathing alone in a candle-lit bathroom, the experience can be extremely relaxing, especially if you have added to your water 3 drops of lavender and 3 drops of neroli essential oils. If you are inviting your lover to share your candle-lit bath, then add 2 drops of sandalwood to the blend to increase its sensuality.

Light candles and a scent burner to transform a living room into a haven of peace after a busy day. Placed in one corner like a perfumed altar, they will bring a feeling of serenity into a room. For a special effect, place a row of candles in front of a mantelpiece mirror to create a beautiful sparkle of reflected light. A single candle, burning quietly in one area of your kitchen, will purify the air and turn the scene of your everyday chores into a more sensual setting. When the heart is disturbed or the mind under stress, sit quietly and gaze at the steady flame of a candle to regain a feeling of peace and repose. If this is combined with the aromatic effects of nature's essential oils, placed in a scent-burner or anointed onto the body from a suitable blend, then the soothing, calming benefits will penetrate very deep.

Nowadays, there are many different types of candles and candle holders to choose from. Go to a special candle shop or to a craft show and take your pick. Choose your candles to suit different moods and occasions. Pick red candles for passion and festive events; green for earthy sensuality; blue, lilac, and pink for romance and love; or white for peace and meditation.

SCENTING YOUR LINGERIE

Using essential oils to fragrance your lingerie is a wonderful way to enhance your own sense of freshness or sexy seductiveness, and may certainly produce a tantalizing effect on your partner. You may choose to add a certain aroma to all your clothes, or perfume only your lingerie as a fragrant surprise for your lover. Imagine how sensual it is to remove your outer clothing to reveal the scent of a delicate flower or a bouquet of exotic blooms. Your lingerie is an intimate and very personal part of your wardrobe, for it is worn close to your skin and often reflects the sensual image you have of yourself. You should always store your lingerie with care, arranging the practical, comfortable pieces in one place, and the soft, silky luxurious items somewhere else. Then you can pick or change your underwear with ease to reflect your mood or the occasion. In that way, you will be able to match your scents with your style of lingerie, for some will be better suited to the aroma of fresh spring flowers, while other pieces should definitely exude a more erotic odor.

It is extremely important, however, not to put the essential oils into a washing machine or any place where they have direct contact with your clothing, as their potent properties can easily stain material. A quick and easy method of perfuming your underwear is to add 2 to 3 drops of essential oil to a few cotton balls. Make sure that the oil has soaked into the cotton before placing it in your lingerie drawer. This will be particularly effective if the drawer is in safe but close proximity to a heater or radiator. Alternatively, you can add a hot-water bottle to your drawer to quicken the evaporation of the oil and scent your clothes.

For a more lasting fragrance, cut up some attractive wallpaper to fit your drawer. Then take 2 cotton balls, and this time add 5 drops of essential oils to them. Rub the back of the wallpaper with your scented cotton balls, and then place the sheets of paper in the bottom of your drawer.

Perhaps you would prefer to use the flowers and herbs themselves to perfume your lingerie. You may choose to combine a variety of herbs and flowers or even roots. Fresh jasmine or lavender, or sweet-scented rose petals, will add a particularly wonderful aroma to your favorite pieces. You can combine the fresh, uplifting scent of lavender with a small amount of spicy chopped gingerroot or mix together romantic jasmine with sexy, stimulating basil. Place your flowers or herbs in a cheesecloth bag and tuck them away in your drawer to infuse your delicate clothing with their lovely smells.

If you are seeking a seductive recipe of essential oils for your lingerie drawer, then blend together 2 drops of neroli for its haunting sweet fragrance with 1 drop of heady, exotic jasmine. For a delightful fresh flowery smell, mix 3 drops of lavender with 2 drops of bergamot. To add zest and a touch of exotic perfume to your underclothes, choose to blend 3 drops of warm, spicy black pepper, 2 drops of sweet ylang ylang, and 1 drop of lime. Men can also enhance the aroma of their underwear, choosing the more woody or masculine scents of sandalwood, jasmine, and orange. Use one drop of each to create a warm and sensual fragrance.

It is always so refreshing when clothes are naturally scented by flowers, spices, and herbs. You can capture their fragrances by sewing small quantities of them into a bag or even buying flower bags from a shop. By following the simple recipes given here, or making up your own, you can perfume your clothes racks, closets, drawers, cupboards, towels, drying racks, and pillows. Also you can take the beautiful smell with you whenever you travel, by putting lavender bags into your suitcase. Or put a lavender and dried ginger bag in your office drawer so whenever you open it you can enjoy its fresh, spicy aroma, bringing to you a moment of pleasure and relaxation. To be really practical, slip your scented bags into your shoes to deodorize them and keep your feet sweet-smelling.

To make your own bags, mix the lavender or other flowers, herbs, and spices to create the perfect scent by which to gently perfume your clothes, or use them to put in certain rooms of your house. Then place your floral or spicy mixtures in gauze or cheesecloth bags and then sew up. Add a drop or two of essential oil to these bags before you seal them. For the bedroom, you may want to add some lavender and geranium drops to your scented bags to exude a feeling of peace and balance. To keep summery clothes like silks and linens smelling cool, hang a bag on your rod containing peppermint leaves (use fresh peppermint, or takes the leaves from a tea bag), and mix together with some refreshing dried lemon peel. Enhance the lovely citrus smell with an uplifting drop of bergamot essential oil. For cool weather clothes, such as sweaters and jackets, introduce a warming smell. You can choose from marjoram, lavender, rosemary, and spicy ginger.

Before you hang your scented bags among your clothes, take a little extra time to beautify your racks and closets. A little "spring-cleaning" of your clothes and wardrobe can bring unexpected rewards. The energy that you put into your clothes is an external reflection of the care that you take of yourself. Throw away clothes that you no longer wear or like. Organize your closet so it is visually pleasing to the eye as well as being an aromatic joy. One idea is to create a color scheme, putting together first all your white clothes, then those that are cream, then yellows, reds, pinks, mauves, purples, blues, and so on. Or you may choose to arrange them by texture, keeping your winter woolens together, and your silks and satins in another part. That way it will be easier to choose the perfect scents for the appropriate clothes.

The aroma of bags will only last a short time, so take care to renew them after the smell has gone.

FOR YOUR SCENTED KITCHEN BAGS

Herbaceous
Mix lavender flowers with dried rosemary for a wonderful herbaceous perfume.

Cure-all
Rosemary has been used over the centuries as a cure-all. It dispels gloom and actually keeps mice and insects at bay.

Woodland
Perhaps, instead, you would like to introduce the smell of the forest into your home. You can pick and dry the woodland debris, making a cheesecloth bag of pine needles mixed with oak moss and adding to it a drop of cedarwood oil.

ARRANGING
FLOWERS

Men and women have always had a love affair with flowers, for they gladden our hearts as surely as their radiant or delicate hues appeal to the eye and their exquisite perfumes delight our sense of smell. Long before the renewed popularity of aromatic essential oils, many of which are distilled from fragrant petals, people have arranged flowers about their home or grown them in pots and window boxes to bathe in the benediction of their colors, sensual shapes, and scents. The appeal of flowers is ancient and worldwide.

Flowers come in so many varieties of color, shape and texture, with a little practice you can learn to arrange your own floral bouquets to adorn your home. The pleasure and beauty they bring will be enhanced by the presence of a lighted candle or an aromatherapy burner, but do make sure that your essential oils complement the fragrance of the flowers. You can choose your blooms to match your mood or to reflect the current season. Certain flowers suit particular rooms and do much to create a special ambience.

For instance, bright, uplifting daffodils look wonderful in the kitchen and dining room, and will herald the return of spring. They can also be planted in boxes to cheer up any windowsill with their yellow trumpet flowers. The refreshing citrus smell of bergamot oil in your scent burner will capture their spirit completely.

A sprig of blossom in your living or bedroom will give it a

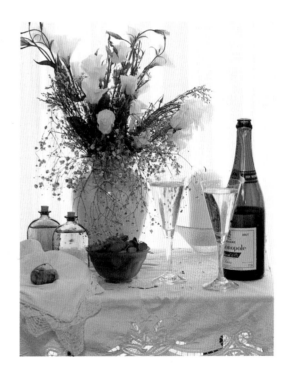

A BEAUTIFUL ARRANGEMENT OF

FLOWERS WILL LIFT THE SPIRITS

graceful and delicate feel. Choose cherry blossom, the flower so loved in Japan, and held in high esteem as a symbol of purity and romance. Or display pinkish-white apple blossom to add a touch of magic, for this was the bough carried by the fairy folk in ancient Celtic tales. Choose haunting bittersweet neroli, the orange blossom perfume, together with a few drops of sandalwood if you wish to light your scent burner.

Roses, of course, are the flowers of the heart, transforming any room into a temple of love. Arrange them in a beautiful vase, and on the opposite side of the room burn 5 drops of rose oil in your scent burner. Your home will soon smell like Cleopatra's palace. The color of roses has some significance, too. Red roses are for deep and everlasting love; cream roses symbolize pure love; while yellow roses may reveal that someone is feeling jealous.

Lilies are the flower of silence and will bring a feeling of peace to your bedroom or lounge. Arrange the tall stalks and flowers in an elegant vase, and then use a white altar candle to soften your room with a mellow glow. Lilies also represent purity and are used in services of worship. They are perfectly complemented by the spiritually uplifting perfume of frankincense. Place 5 drops of the essential oil in an aromatherapy burner to add the essence of meditation to your environment.

Orchids bring the warm, lush Orient into your home. Place a few drops of ylang ylang, black pepper, and orange into your scent burner to enhance their sense of the exotic.

SCENT BURNERS

Scent burners are an essential tool in the art of aromatherapy and play a particularly important role in creating a sensual ambience. They are by far the best way of introducing essential oils into the atmosphere, thus affecting our emotions directly as well as emitting their special blend of fragrances.

The growing popularity of aromatherapy means that burners are now easily available from specialist shops, craft shows and many markets. They can come in many shapes and may be made of glass, ceramics, or terracotta, among other materials. It is worthwhile spending a little extra money to buy a burner which is beautifully designed. Look for one that has a pot large enough to hold a sufficient quantity of water to allow your oils to evaporate into the air over a longer period of time. The distance between the bottom of the pot and the lighted candle should be enough so that the water remains hot but never boils.

Aromatherapy burners can be used throughout the house, though it is probably unwise to have more than two burners of different perfumes alight at any one time. The whole point of aromatics is that the specific properties of the oils have a chance to work on the body, mind, and emotions. Too many conflicting smells will confuse the olfactory senses and even lead to a feeling of nausea.

By studying the essential oil profiles in chapter 1 and by reading the recipes given throughout this book, you will become familiar with different oils and their benefits. You can follow the recipes given in this book, or you can begin to make up your own blends.

Scent is a very personal choice, and slowly you will begin to recognize those perfumes which are special to you. Up to 7 drops of a combination of any 3 oils can be used in a burner at any one time. For as long as the burner is filled with water, the aromatics should be working their spell.

AROMATHERAPY BURNERS AND CANDLES TRANSFORM ANY ROOM

A scent burner plays a particularly useful role if you need a change in atmosphere, for example, if you have moved, changed job, or just ended a relationship. A blend of 3 drops of juniper, 2 drops clary sage, and 2 drops sandalwood will purify and cleanse old vibrations and allow the new to emerge.

Six drops of bergamot placed into the burner will act as a deodorant, clearing a room of the smell of smoke or food. To fill your home with the essence of love, burn 2 drops of sandalwood combined with 4 drops of rose. You can also light candles and fill your vases with roses of cream and red to add to the overall effects of your burner. Or at the end of the day when you need to relax, put 4 drops of lavender and 3 drops jasmine into the burner to take you away from the cares of the world.

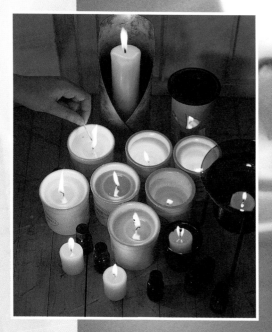

Aromatherapy burners should not be left unattended, especially if children or pets are in the room. Their presence in your home, though, will add much to its esthetics and comfort, so that after a while, it will be almost impossible to imagine being there without the subtle background fragrance of nature's beautiful gifts.

SCENTING YOUR
BED LINEN

There could be few things more romantic than being seduced on a bed strewn with fragrant flower petals. They could be spread over the top cover as a carpet of love, or hidden below the sheet to be exposed in all their perfumed glory as you are taken into the bed. Perhaps those petals have been arranged in the shape of a heart or some other significant design as they nestle upon the pillow. Even more enticing would be to find a trail of petals or flowers leading from the front door to the bedroom along which you could be led toward your love den. As a woman, you could create an even more tantalizing, if less subtle pathway to paradise, by scattering en route your sexiest items of lingerie. Imagine if this impossibly romantic setting was softly illuminated by candlelight, and perfumed with the aroma of erotic essential oils from a scent burner which complemented perfectly the fragrance of the flowers – then certainly it would be a night to remember forever.

You could choose to create this beautiful scene to delight and surprise your partner on a special anniversary or simply to bring the romance back into your love life. Pick flower petals which are soft and sensual to touch and which add to the tactile feel of the bed. Any fragrant flower can be used, though jasmine, orange blossom, or lime blossom would make an excellent choice for their exotic, alluring, or playful qualities. There is no doubt, however, that roses are by far the most romantic of flowers and have always been the most popular floral choice of lovers. Just like the legend of Cleopatra and Mark Anthony, you could surrender to love on a bed of roses. The fragrance of the rose petals would uplift and open your hearts, and cling to your skin like fragments of silk.

To create such a sensual ambience as the one just described is something you would do for purely memorable occasions. Yet there are many practical ways you can keep your bed linen fragrant and fresh to add that extra allure to your time of rest, sleep, or love-making. When drying your sheets and covers, put an absorbent cloth, such as a washcloth, on which you have placed 4 to 5 drops of essential oil, into the dryer, or hang small bags of fresh flowers, spices, and herbs along your drying rack, to infuse their aroma into the linen. Finally, you can store your clean, folded sheets in the linen cupboard, with cotton pads impregnated with essential oils placed close by.

You can even blend your oils to impregnate your sheets with special scents which will lull you into a deep sleep, give you sweet dreams, enhance a night of love, or make you feel fresh and clean.

To help you sleep deeply, put 2 drops of chamomile and 3 drops of lavender essential oils on the cotton pads. Both those oils will bring about a feeling of calm and ease. For sweet dreams, choose 2 drops of clary sage and 3 drops of neroli. A sensual night could be spent between sheets smelling sweetly of heart-opening rose and warming black pepper – add 3 drops of rose with 2 drops of black pepper. Sometimes, to climb between crisp fresh sheets is very appealing, especially if you or a member of your family is ill. Use 2 drops of bergamot and 2 drops of pine essential oil.

CREATING A BEAUTIFUL BATHROOM

Too often the importance of the bathroom as a place of cleansing, purification, and refuge of the body and mind is overlooked. It is a room that is worthy of receiving your most creative thoughts and should be as ambient a setting as your bedroom. Even if your bathroom is small, there are many little touches that will make a difference. By beautifying this room, you are creating a place where you can completely relax and unwind, washing away the tensions of the day, or preparing yourself for a special date or a night of pleasure.

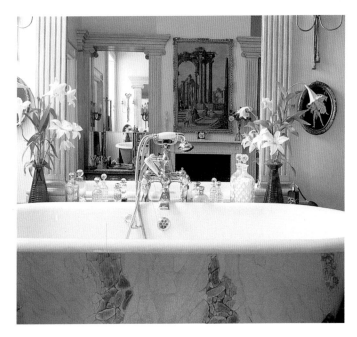

You may want to put some plants in your bathroom – ferns look inviting and will grow well in the moist environment. Keep beautiful colored glass bottles on a shelf to glitter like jewels in candlelight. In these bottles you can store your aromatic essential oils. Blend a number of recipes for different occasions, mixing up to 15 drops of the essentials oils with 5tsp of base oil. Choose a green bottle for a refreshing, invigorating, and stimulating mix of oils. Fill your blue bottles with the relaxing blends, and select red bottles for aphrodisiac and sensual recipes for whenever you invite your lover to join you in the bath, or plan a pampering evening just for yourself.

YOUR BATHROOM CAN BECOME A REFUGE OF BEAUTY AND SENSUALITY

There may be many ways to make your bathroom more

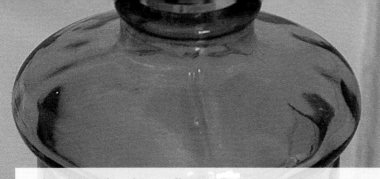

welcoming. Color always affects our senses; check to see if your towels, curtains, and mats are harmonious. Blue and green are the colors of healing and beauty, and are especially suitable to the bathroom, though a splash of red here and there will add a touch of passion. Sea shells are perfect as ornaments in a bathroom and instill a sense of watery, oceanic bliss. Throw away old cosmetics and keep only those which feel and smell good to you and are kind to your skin. Choose to use beautiful scented soaps that are perfumed with essential oils, and always keep a loofah nearby to stimulate and invigorate your skin. Try using sea sponges, which have a soothing texture.

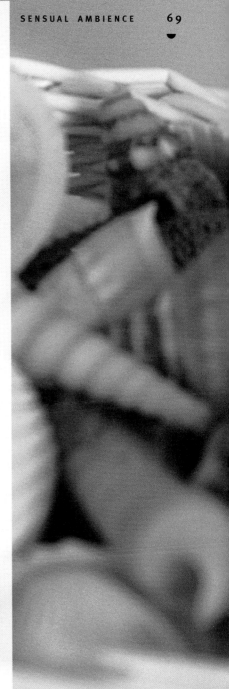

While you soak in the bath, you may want to burn some oils in an aromatherapy burner and simply lie back to inhale the scent, letting your cares drop away from you in the steaming warmth of the water. Consult the essential oil profiles at the beginning of the book to choose your oils, depending on whatever mood you wish to enhance. Up to 7 drops of essential oils can be put in a scent burner or into a bath. For a bathing ritual, place some fresh cut flowers in the bathroom and light some soft blue candles. Make sure that you have warm, softly scented towels to wrap yourself in when you step out of the bath. Then as you lie in the water, perform a simple exercise. Be aware of your body, and begin to consciously release the tensions out of every muscle. Focus first on your legs and feet, and travel up your body. Then consciously allow every part of you to absorb the healing energies of the oils.

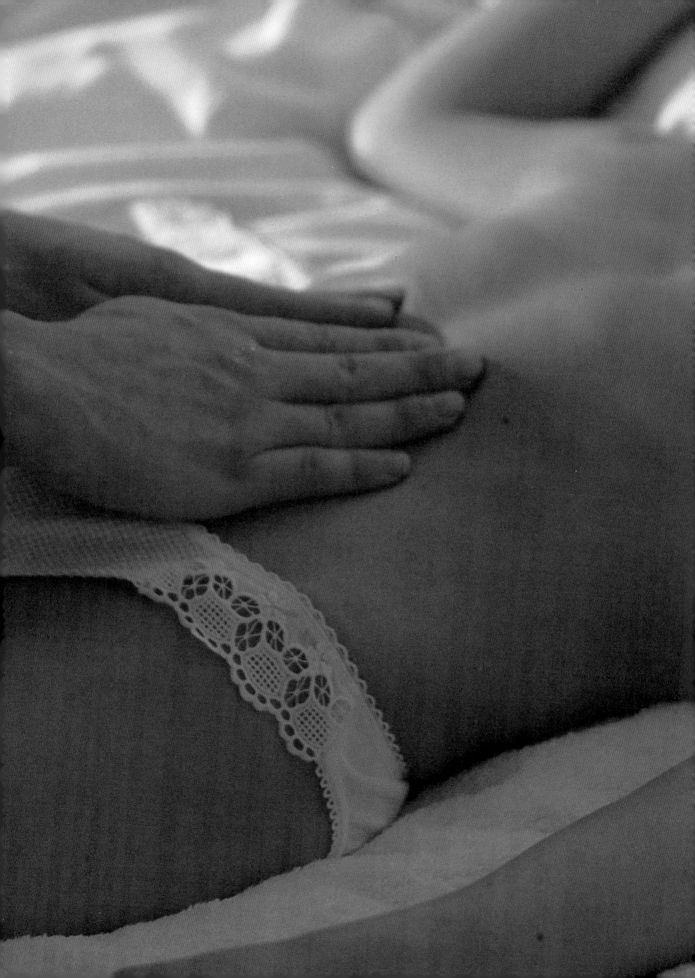

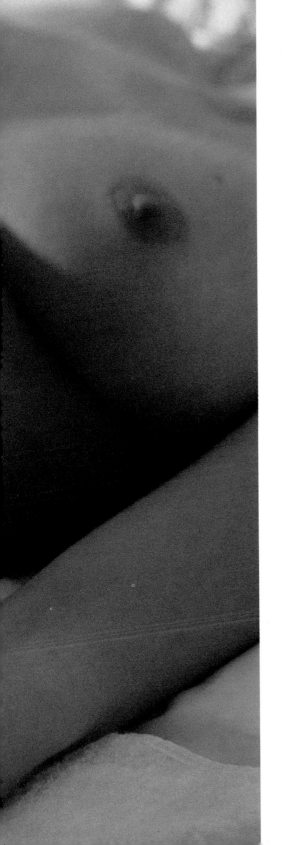

therapeutic massage

The combination of aromatic essential oils with massage is a marriage made in heaven. Both are functions of natural healing, restoring balance to the body and mind, and bringing about a sense of well-being. Aromatherapy massage can help both you and your partner to enhance your relationship in many ways – emotionally, physically, and spiritually. In the following chapter, you will learn about oil recipes and strokes of massage to pamper your loved one, release stress, and invigorate. You will discover that an essential oil massage can be an indulgent, euphoric and deeply relaxing experience, or one that is sensually, emotionally and sexually enlivening. You will learn, too, how important the senses in our skin are in increasing and heightening our awareness. To set the scene for massage, study the suggestions in Chapter 3. It is always a good idea before giving a massage to make sure the room is heated. Add to the atmosphere with candles, bowls of potpourri, and flowers.

Blend your oils according to your selected recipe, but check Chapter 1 to see if any are contra-indicated. Always take special care when using bergamot. If you have blended this oil in a recipe to use on your skin, make sure you do not expose yourself to the sun or ultraviolet light as it increases photosensitivity. Use one recipe at a time if you intend to give a whole-body massage – the effects will be profound whether you massage a part or all of the body.

A MASSAGE TO
pamper

RECIPES FOR A PAMPERING MASSAGE

RECIPE 1

Pampering and Devotion

Lavender, Geranium, Rose

For Face and Head Massage

To 2tsp base oil combining 1tsp each of jojoba and sweet almond add:

2 drops Lavender

1 drop Geranium

2 drops Rose

For Whole Body Massage

To 5tsp base oil of equal jojoba and sweet almond mix add:

5 drops Lavender

3 drops Geranium

5 drops Rose

When you love someone, there are times when you simply want to stretch out to caress them, or to take away their stress or pain with a tender touch. Instinctively, you know that making contact in this way can be very healing and soothing. Whenever you want to pamper your partner, to share with him or her the care and devotion you feel, or to stroke away tension and uplift the spirit, what could be better than to offer to give a face and head massage? You may spend only between twenty to thirty minutes on the massage, but its effects, when combined with the relaxing and luxuriant properties of the essential oils, will help to remedy stress, calm the mind, and reassure your partner of your devotion. If you blend the essential oils from the first recipe, using lavender, geranium, and the ever-lovely rose, their calming, nurturing, and balancing properties mean she feels cherished and deeply relaxed.

If you sense she is anxious or needs a boost to her energy, then you may want, instead, to blend the essences of frankincense, bergamot, and jasmine into the basic oil mix to leave her feeling inspired and uplifted. The special properties of the sweet almond and jojoba base oil mix will also nurture her skin.

Whichever recipe you choose, she will be comforted, not only by the healing aromas, but also by the caring quality of touch in your hands. Few things can be more intimate than a tender face massage. Sit or kneel behind your partner and make sure that you are comfortably supported by pillows. She can then rest her head close to your lap. When you massage the face, make sure that your hands apply a steady but sensitive pressure, flowing smoothly from one area to another. Spread the tiny amount of oil over her throat and face, with soft, sweeping strokes that yield to her facial contours.

To relax her jaw, cup your hands over each side of it, so your fingertips meet on her chin. Rest them lightly in this position for up to sixty seconds. Let the still, warmth of your touch melt away muscle tightness. Then caress her face by sweeping each hand, one after the other up over her jaw several times, lifting them away as they reach just below her ears. Press and gently squeeze along the rims of her ears, then stroke behind them. With relaxed hands, circulate your fingertips smoothly over both cheeks. Lightly sweep the first two fingers of each hand around the bony circumference of each eye five times. Never put pressure on the eyes directly or drag on the delicate skin below them.

Softly cup your hands to her head, and stroke both thumbs steadily out from the center of her brow to the sides of her head. Repeat so that your thumbs stroke outward, line by line, over the entire surface of her forehead. Soothe her temples by circulating your fingertips over them. Complete with a scalp massage and then lovingly comb your fingers through her hair.

TO FINISH, MAKE FIRM FINGERTIP CIRCLES

RECIPE 2

Uplifting and Calming
Frankincense, Bergamot,*
Jasmine
(*Note Bergamot caution on previous page)

For Face and Head Massage
To 2tsp base oil combine 1tsp each of jojoba and sweet almond and add:
2 drops Frankincense,
1 drop Bergamot
2 drops Jasmine

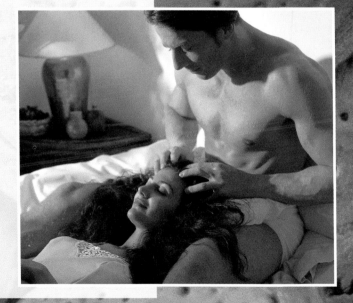

ease stress

SHOULDERS AND NECK

The shoulder and neck region is the area of the body most inclined to gather tension from everyday stress, emotional upset, or bad posture. Most people have experienced, from time to time, discomfort or stiffness in this area and the accompanying aches and pains. This part of the body is prone to tighten when we feel ourselves overwhelmed by emotions such as anger and anxiety, suffer work and domestic stress, or are simply frustrated by every day occurrences such as being caught in a traffic jam. Sitting for prolonged periods at a desk or computer, or moving the body in the wrong way, can also lead to muscular tension in the top of the back. If the tensions are not released, the contracted muscles restrict the blood flow to the head and brain, causing headaches and making us feel tired and irritable.

A fifteen-minute shoulder, neck, and head massage can work wonders to alleviate these symptoms. If you recognize your partner's stress signals, you can offer him a shoulder rub and put him in a better mood. By applying a few easy strokes and trusting in the relaxing and caring quality of your touch, you and your partner can respond lovingly to each other's tensions, helping to ease away the pain and returning one another to good humor.

To enhance the beneficial effect of your massage, use either recipe shown on this page to add some essences to your base oil. Clary sage, sandalwood, and ylang ylang all help to release emo-

RECIPES FOR A MASSAGE TO EASE STRESS

RECIPE 1
Releasing Stress
Clary Sage, Jasmine, Sandalwood

For Shoulder and Neck Massage
To 1tbs grapeseed and sunflower base oil mix add:
2 drops Clary Sage
2 drops Jasmine
4 drops Sandalwood

For Whole Body Massage
To 1tbs base oil mix add:
4 drops Clary Sage
4 drops Jasmine
6 drops Sandalwood

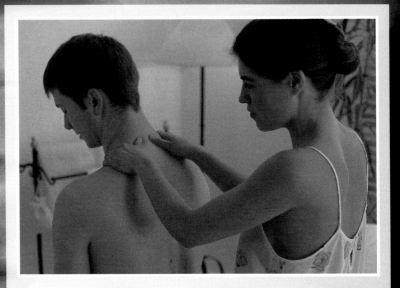

MASSAGING THE BACK AND NECK CAN RELIEVE EVERYDAY TENSION

tional and physical tensions and to relax the mind. Jasmine, ginger, and black pepper add warmth and stimulation, loosening stiff joints.

Have your partner sit comfortably In front of you. Place some oil into the palms of your hands and spread it with flowing strokes over the upper back and neck, and across the shoulders and tops of the arms. Place both hands flat between his shoulders, and slide them firmly up between them before fanning out to the tops of the arms and down the sides of his rib cage. Glide back to the original position and repeat several times. Hook your fingers over the shoulders and use your thumbs to make small circles into the tight areas along the spine and up around the shoulder blades. Massage the neck, gently squeezing the muscles between the fingers and thumb of your other hand. For an enlivening finish, pummel his shoulders and tease the skin with light strokes.

RECIPE 2

Warming and Relaxing

Ginger, Black Pepper,
Ylang Ylang

For Shoulder and
Neck Massage

To 1tbs grapeseed and
sunflower oil add:

3 drops Ginger
3 drops Black Pepper
2 drops Ylang Ylang

For Whole Body
Massage

To 5tsp base oil
mix add:

5 drops Ginger
5 drops Black pepper
4 drops Ylang Ylang

invigoration

RECIPES FOR A MASSAGE FOR INVIGORATION

RECIPE 1

Invigoration

Cedarwood, Black Pepper, Orange

For Back and Buttocks

Massage

To 4tsp base oil mix of
grapeseed and sunflower or
grapeseed and
sweet almond add:

3 drops Cedarwood

4 drops Black Pepper

4 drops Orange

For Whole Body

Massage

To 5tsp mix of the above

mentioned

base oil add:

4 drops Cedarwood

5 drops Black Pepper

5 drops Orange

Regular aromatherapy massage can replenish your physical resources and counteract the negative toll that stress, overwork, and worry can have on your physical and emotional states and consequently, on your relationship. It can restore balance and relaxation to the body and mind, while at the same time boosting the whole physiological system, invigorating the muscles and circulatory system to give you a feeling of renewed energy and vitality.

The three essential oil recipes recommended in this section on massage for invigoration have been carefully selected for their warming, boosting, and restorative properties. Check their specific properties in the plant profiles to choose the appropriate recipe to meet your own or your partner's needs. A twenty-minute back massage, or a sixty-minute whole body massage should help either of you to feel restored and re-energized after a tiring and stressful day, or after a period of low spirits and vitality.

THE BACK MASSAGE

Before giving the massage, check that the room is warm enough, and that your partner is lying comfortably on a firm and supportive mattress. Kneel beside him and start to spread your blended oils over the surface and sides of his back and buttocks. Before employing more invigorating strokes, warm and relax the body's tissues with flowing movements, using the flat of your hands to fan, stretch and circle over his skin at a steady, rhythmic pressure, molding them

to his body's contours. Then straddling his thighs, perform a main

back stroke, repeating up to five times as one continuous motion.

Place your hands flat on each side of the base of his spine, so your

fingers point toward his head.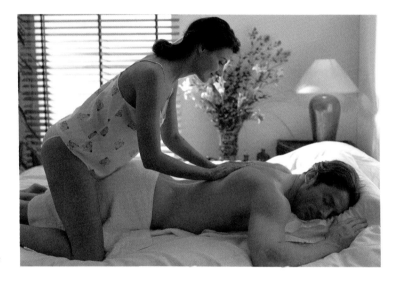
Stroke them steadily upward in
one long motion toward the
shoulders to give a satisfying
and relaxing stretch to the muscles and ligaments surrounding
the vertebrae. Fan both hands
firmly out to the shoulder joints,
creating a good stretch to the
muscles surrounding the base of

the neck. Lean your body back as you mold and pull your hands **THE INVIGORATING OIL AND YOUR**

down along the sides of the rib cage, turning them at the base of **STROKES RELIEVE HIS STRESS**

the back to glide them toward their starting position.

To help boost the blood flow toward the heart, perform a

series of smaller, interweaving fan-shaped strokes that move up

along the back. Slide both hands as before upward for about six

inches, then glide them out to enfold both sides of the body. Pull

back down and then, by flicking your wrists, turn them around to

return to the source of the stroke. Repeat the movement without

pausing, sliding the stroke to a higher level of the back. At the top

of the back, widen the fanning motion to encircle the shoulders

RECIPE 2
Enlivening and Playful
Lime, Basil, Bergamot

For Back and Buttocks Massage
To 4tsp base oil mix of
grapeseed and sunflower or
grapeseed and
sweet almond add:
5 drops Lime
4 drops Basil
3 drops Bergamot

For Whole Body Massage
To a 5tsp mix of above
mentioned
base oils add:
6 drops Lime
5 drops Basil
4 drops Bergamot

before gliding your hands back as before to their original position. Repeat the sequence several times, building up speed, pressure, and tempo to increase the invigorating effects.

Before you start the kneading strokes, focus more attention on the spine. Press your thumb pads into the grooves, each side of the lower end of the spine, with your hands resting on his body, relaxed and at an angle. Slide your thumbs firmly alongside the spinal column toward the shoulder blades. Then sweep your hands over the upper back and shoulders, returning them to the base of the back as in previous strokes. Repeat the stretch twice.

Hands and oils are now working together to replenish vital energy and boost the body's physiological systems. If you are using Recipe 1 shown on the previous page, the combined essences of cedarwood, black pepper, and orange will be working their magic on your partner while your strokes unlock his tensions. Cedarwood

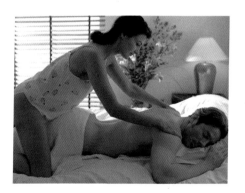

provides an all-round tonic for his system and increases mental alertness, while black pepper adds spice and warmth to ease stiff muscles. The essence

FAN YOUR HANDS OUTWARD

of orange gives zest and energy, cleansing the blood and detoxifying the skin while also soothing muscular aches and loosening their tightness.

Perhaps you have chosen, instead, to blend the essences from Recipe 2, shown on this page, to restore his vitality. The lime replenishes vital resources, tones and refreshes, and works as a digestive stimulant, while basil strengthens the central nervous system, enhancing the positive effects of the spinal stretch strokes, while also relieving physical and mental fatigue. The bergamot uplifts the spirits, eases depression, and encourages the appetite. Recipe 3, shown on the next page, combines the warm and stimulating properties of ginger with the cheerful, tangy effects of orange.

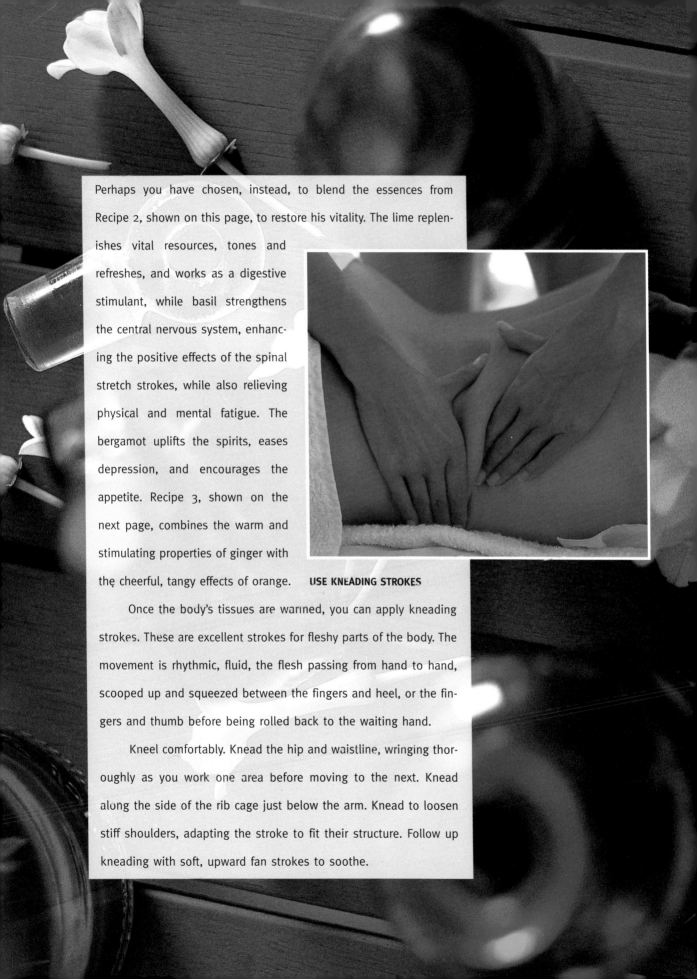

USE KNEADING STROKES

Once the body's tissues are warmed, you can apply kneading strokes. These are excellent strokes for fleshy parts of the body. The movement is rhythmic, fluid, the flesh passing from hand to hand, scooped up and squeezed between the fingers and heel, or the fingers and thumb before being rolled back to the waiting hand.

Kneel comfortably. Knead the hip and waistline, wringing thoroughly as you work one area before moving to the next. Knead along the side of the rib cage just below the arm. Knead to loosen stiff shoulders, adapting the stroke to fit their structure. Follow up kneading with soft, upward fan strokes to soothe.

THE BUTTOCKS MASSAGE

SOFT STROKES ON THE BUTTOCKS WILL WARM THE MUSCLES AND SKIN

Once the back is relaxed but tingling with vitality, turn your attention and strokes to his buttocks. Most men enjoy receiving an invigorating massage on this area, finding it stimulating on both a physical and a sensual level. By relieving muscular tension in the lower back, buttocks, and thighs, you can alleviate strain throughout the whole body, bringing greater ease to his overall posture and movement. Also, the buttocks are a highly erotic zone of the body, with large, strong muscles amply supplied with sensory nerves that increase responsiveness in the pelvis and genital area. A sensual and invigorating buttocks massage combined with the warming and stimulating essential oils recommended in this section will not only relax any muscular tension, but may also put him back in the mood for making love.

Begin by relaxing and warming the buttocks with some soft and flowing strokes, softening your hands so they sculpt and shape his sensual curves. Kneel to one side of his thighs, and spread the essential oil mix over the skin, sweeping both hands over the surface and sides of the buttocks in a spiraling circular motion. Include the lower back and tops of the thighs in your strokes. Then turning to face toward his head, slide both hands, little fingers leading, over the top of his thighs to enfold the swell of his buttocks. Fan both hands out over the crest of his pelvis to sweep past the hips, sliding them back to the upper thighs. Turn your wrists to repeat the stroke several times as one continuous and unbroken motion.

The strong muscles in this region can withstand a firm pressure once the area has become relaxed by your more sensual strokes. To knead over the buttocks, you may need to swap your position to work on the opposite side. Knead firmly but in a fluid d motion all over the buttocks, lifting the flesh in one hand, then squeezing and rolling it back and forth between both hands. This fleshy area is simply perfect for the thoroughly satisfying effects of the kneading stroke. Take the stroke down to the upper thigh, kneading thoroughly over its surface and sides. Then soothe the whole area by repeating the sensual movements wilh which you staited the buttocks massage.

For a stimulating finish to the buttock massage, apply some percussion strokes that will tone the muscles, and enliven the skin. Then tease the skin with light feathery strokes.

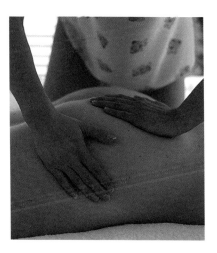

THE WARMING EFFECT OF GINGER AND ORANGE WILL ENHANCE YOUR STROKES

RECIPE 3
Warming and Uplifting
Ginger, Orange

For Back and Buttocks
Massage
To 4tsp base oil mix of
grapeseed and sunflower or
grapeseed and
sweet almond add:
4 drops Ginger
5 drops Orange

For Whole Body
Massage
To 5tsp of above mentioned
base oil mix add:
5 drops Ginger
6 drops Orange

A MASSAGE FOR
pure relaxation

RECIPES FOR A MASSAGE FOR PURE RELAXATION

RECIPE 1

Euphoric

Clary Sage,
Frankincense, Lime

For Legs and Feet
Massage

To 2tsp base oil mix of
safflower, sunflower, grapeseed, or sweet
almond add:
2 drops Clary Sage
1 drop Frankincense
3 drops Lime

For Whole Body
Massage

To base oil mix of
ingredients mentioned
above add:
5 drops Clary Sage
3 drops Frankincense

Imagine how blissful it would be, if at the end of the day, your partner treated you to a luxurious massage for pure relaxation. He has taken the time to create an inviting and sensual ambience for the occasion. The room has been warmed, and flickering candles cast a romantic and soporific glow over the scene. Vases of delicate flowers delight your eye. The mattress is covered with fresh, warm sheets or towels, and pillows are scattered on it for you to lie back comfortably. Soft music is playing in the background. The air is fragrant with the aroma of blended essential oils, perhaps filled with the haunting, resinous smell of frankincense, the perfume of the gods; or the deeply floral odor of bright geranium. Maybe he has chosen jasmine, the sacred flower of the East, to seduce your olfactory senses with its exquisite exotic smell and combined it with the refreshingly citric and flowery fragrance of bergamot.

Receiving a massage to the legs and feet is very relaxing, stroking away the weariness from sore muscles in the calves and thighs and removing strain from the tendons and ligaments of the feet. The upward flowing strokes boost the blood circulation toward the heart and aid the flow of lymph toward the lymph glands, helping your immune system to eliminate toxins from the body.

As he leads you to the room to lie back into the pillows, all of your senses feel alive and heightened. Now is the time to wallow in the sensual pleasure of being given a loving massage on your legs and feet. His tender strokes will be enhanced by the beneficial properties of the essential oils, which will nourish your skin and uplift and lighten you both physically and emotionally. A leg and feet massage, by itself, can be enough to seduce your mind into a state of euphoria. If he chooses to give you a whole body massage, it will be ecstasy indeed! Let this fantasy become a reality within your relationship, so that on different occasions, you find the time to surprise and pleasure each other, asking no more than to be given the opportunity to offer to your loved one the gift of a luxurious massage.

THE LEG MASSAGE

Rub some oil into your palms, and spread it down one leg at a time with overlapping strokes. Let your hands be gentle in touch, molding to the shape of the legs. Then let your hands flow freely and smoothly over both legs, inducing warmth and vitality, always rounding off your strokes. Remember, never to conclude your strokes abruptly. Now focus on one leg, gliding both hands steadily up its whole length, shaping them softly over the knee and fanning them out at the top of her thigh to cup the

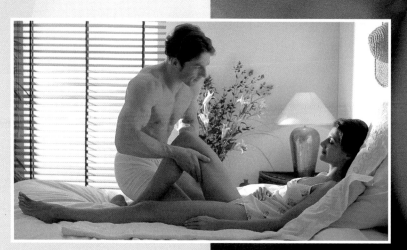

sides of the leg. Without breaking the motion, slip your fingers

---

RECIPE 2

Let go

Cedarwood, Geranium

For Legs and Feet Massage

To 2tsp base oil mix of safflower, grapeseed or sweet almond add:

4 drops Cedarwood

2 drops Bergamot

For Whole Body Massage

To 5tsp of above mentioned base oil mix add:

8 drops Cedarwood

6 drops Geranium

behind the thigh and pull gently but steadily downward till your hands glide out over her foot. This will give her leg a lovely, relaxing stretch. Repeat this long stroke several times as a continuous flow so your hands feel like molten liquid washing over her skin. Then fan your hands, one motion softly looping into the other over the leg to the top of her thighs, before gliding them back down as before. Cover the sensual and erogenous area of her thigh with flowing motions, fan and circle strokes, and then knead if this stroke feels appropriate. With feather-light touches, trail your fingertips, one hand following the other in over-lapping motions all the way down her leg. Repeat all these strokes on her other leg.

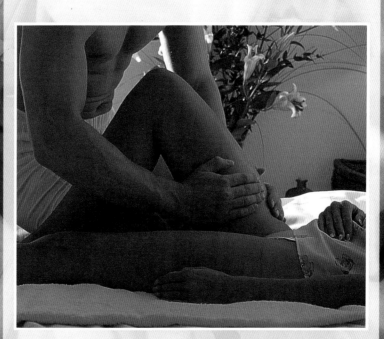

YOUR FLOWING STROKES WILL HELP THE OILS

TO PENETRATE THE SKIN

THE FOOT MASSAGE

A foot massage stimulates the many nerve endings in its sole, giv-

ing a boost to the internal system. Pressing and manipulating the foot gently will ease its tension and enhance its suppleness and mobility. It is, however, the sensual and deeply relaxing qualities of the oils together with the languid caresses of the hands against the skin which induce the luxuriant feelings of lavish indulgence and pure relaxation.

Begin the foot massage with a calming and balancing hold, resting your hands in a still manner over them for up to sixty sec-onds. Then focusing on one foot at a time, spread a little more oil over its surface with flowing strokes. Glide both hands over the instep, then with fingers encircling the ankle bones, draw then out over both sides of the foot. Massage all over the top, sides, and bottom of the foot with your heels, thumbs ,and fingers, supporting the foot with the free hand. Stretch each toe from base to tip

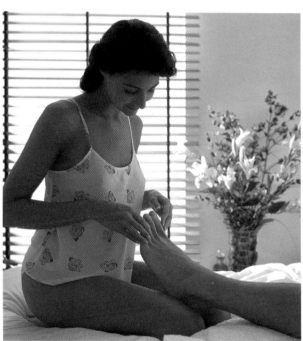

between the thumb and index finger, swapping hands when neces-sary. Feather stroke over the foot to enliven the skin, then cradle it between your palms. Repeat all the strokes on the other foot, fin-ishing with the balancing hold for up to a minute. The warmth of your hands on his feet will be calming.

THE FEET ARE

PARTICULARLY SENSITIVE

TO FEATHERY TOUCHES

A MASSAGE FOR
sexual openness

THE ABDOMEN

Sensual massage, combined with the aphrodisiac qualities of certain essential oils, can enhance sexual feelings and emotional openness between loving partners to enrich their intimacy and spontaneity. When there is mutual consent, aromatic massage can become part of foreplay, a prelude to lovemaking, or it may simply be enjoyed for its own sake – a way of bonding and bringing both people into a caring, loving, and physical closeness.

Choose the woody aroma of juniper essence, combined with earthy sandalwood, to help build trust and sexual openness in a new relationship. Or pick sweet, exotic ylang ylang for its sensual, sexual, and relaxing qualities and add to it a warming touch of spicy black

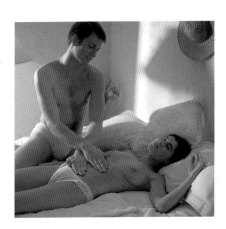

pepper. Give your partner a whole body massage, or focus your strokes on her abdomen and chest, perhaps completing the session with a loving face massage (see page 71).

YOUR STROKES ON HER BELLY SHOULD BE SOFT AND LOVING

The abdomen is a vulnerable and sensitive area, connected closely to our instinctive sexual and emotional feelings. Gentle flowing strokes on this area can relax deep rooted tensions, warm the vital organs, and help your partner breathe more fully so she feels revitalized.

RECIPES FOR A MASSAGE FOR SEXUAL AND EMOTIONAL OPENNESS

RECIPE 1
Emotional Openness
Juniper, Sandalwood

For Abdomen and Chest Massage
To 2tsp base oil mix of jojoba and sweet almond, or grapeseed add:
2 drops *Juniper*
3 drops *Sandalwood*

For Whole Body Massage
To 5tsp base oil mix of above mentioned ingredients add:
5 drops *Juniper*
7 drops *Sandalwood*

Start by facing your partner's abdomen and spread the oil over the front and sides of the body with large circular strokes. Move both hands, with your fingers pointing away from you, in a clockwise motion. Then lift the right hand to let the left hand pass underneath to complete a full circle. Cross the right hand over the left wrist and drop it lightly back onto the abdomen to perform another half-circle motion before lifting off again. Circle the abdomen in this way several times, allowing the muscles to relax and the oils to be absorbed into the skin.

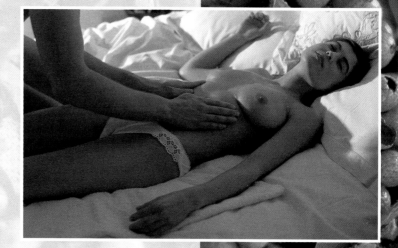

MASSAGE THE CHEST AND STOMACH WITH FRUITY OIL

RECIPE 2

Aphrodisiac
Ylang Ylang, Black Pepper

For Abdomen and
Chest Massage
To 2tsp base oil mix of jojoba
and sweet almond,
or grapeseed add:
2 drops Ylang Ylang
4 drops Black Pepper

Tturn to face your partner's head, and stroke both hands, fingers pointing to the top of the body, up over the surface of the abdomen, before gliding them out to the sides of the rib cage. Continue the stroke, slipping your fingers under her back while molding your hands to her sides. Pull your hands down her waistline and then turn your wrists to let them circle around the hips to their original position. Repeat several times. Face the abdomen, and knead along the opposite side of her body over the hip and waist, repeat on the other side. Perform a few more circle strokes, completing with a still hold. Rest both hands on the abdomen for a minute.

sexual openness

THE CHEST

A loving touch contains both strength and gentleness. Think of the way a mother holds her child, firm enough to impart a sense of reassurance and protection, yet tender and comforting at the same time. This is the quality of caring which should be in your hands as you massage your partner, especially when you stroke the most intimate parts of her body, such as her abdomen, chest, and face. The oils you choose can reflect these qualities, evoking feelings of love, peace, and security.

The third recipe in this section that incorporates strokes on the abdomen and chest suggests a blend of rose and frankincense. This is a beautiful mix of essential oils, combining the aroma of the ultimate flower of love with the meditative properties of the resinous gum. Rose heals the heart, and frankincense brings inner peace while elevating love. If you have chosen this recipe, then its ingredients will reinforce the healing and caring touch of your hands. It is particularly appropriate when applied in a chest massage, for as your strokes embrace this area, they release tensions that protect the inner feelings of vulnerability, sadness, joy, and love that emanate from the heart.

Position yourself behind your partner's head, sitting or kneeling comfortably so you can remain relaxed. Begin with a still hold, placing one hand gently on the crown of her head, and the other lightly over her heart. This calm hold will restore a feeling of balance between mind and body so she is able to let go of anxiety and relax into a sensual frame of mind. Rub some oil into your hands and spread it over her chest and breasts. The following sequence of strokes forms one unbroken motion to warm and loosen tension from the chest and rib cage and expand her breathing. Repeat them several times.

Place both hands flat on the top of her breastbone, fingers pointing down the body. Slide them toward the base of her rib cage, before fanning them out to the sides of her body. Enfold the sides of the ribcage and draw both hands upward with a steady glide. Bringing both hands back onto the

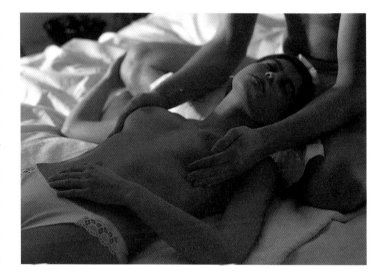

chest above her breasts. Draw them out, heels leading, over the pectorals toward the edges of her shoulders. Encircle her shoulder joints, gliding your hands lightly inward over the back of the shoulders, and then flex the wrists again, to cup her neck securely into the support of your palms. Pull gently but steadily along the back of her neck, and lifting her head slightly, draw your hands out from behind her head. Now perform a series of fanning motions down her chest, one stroke dissolving into the other until your hands glide out and around the base of the rib cage, to return them in the manner of the previous stroke. Cup your hands over her breasts to bring them warmth, then circle softly around them.

IF SHE CONSENTS FOR YOU TO TOUCH HER BREAST, DO SO WITH RESPECT AND GENTLENESS

A MASSAGE TO
heighten skin sensation

RECIPES FOR A MASSAGE TO HEIGHTEN SKIN SENSATION

RECIPE 1
Heightened awareness
Basil, Lavender, Patchouli

For Overall Skin Contact
To 4tsp grapeseed base oil
for a tempting
touch or to 2tsp grapeseed
and 2tsp avocado
or jojoba for
lasting feeling add:
4 drops Basil
4 drops Lavender
2 drops Patchouli

One of the most important aspects of touch is that it brings the senses in our skin alive. It is through our outer layer that we are able to experience and feel all sensation. Skin envelops us and protects us, and it is the meeting point of our external and internal realities. What happens on the outside of the body is transmitted by our feeling senses in the skin to the brain through the central nervous system. The brain then decodes the message and sends its impulses back to the periphery of the body so we are able to respond accordingly. Our skin reflects what happens in our mind, emotions, and feelings – we glow with health and pale with fear; we blush when we are embarrassed and tingle with excitement or we get goose bumps when we are thrilled or frightened. Every inch of the skin is packed with sensory nerve receptors that respond to different tactile stimulation. The skin incorporates our most pervading sense – the sense of touch that functions throughout the entire surface of the body.

Touch, when it comes from another person, affirms to us our self-worth. If we are touched with love, it makes us feel loveable. If we are never touched, we feel isolated and alone. Touch is a form of nourishment, feeding our bodies and minds and keeping us in contact with our innermost feelings.

A healthy and enlivened skin is therefore important to our overall well-being. Nourishing the skin with an essential oil blend and teasing it with loving, playful touches will help to keep it vital and responsive. Choose from one of the recipes shown here and spread the oil lightly over your partner's bare skin, using your palms and fingers to stroke in downward flowing movements. This is not strictly a massage, but more an experience in skin sensation. Then begin to rake your fingertips down over the skin, one hand following the other in overlapping motions. See if she notices the difference in feeling between the pressure of the palms and the raking sensation of the fingertips. Then decrease the pressure even more, tracing the skin with feather touches, focusing them particularly on areas of highly sensitive soft skin. She will feel the nerve endings thrill and tingle to these tantalizing touches. Try the varying pressures on different parts of the body – the palms of the hands, the soles of the feet, the skin of the face, and down the length of the spine. Run your fingertips with the barest touch over her lips, her ears, or the back of her neck.

Some people find this type of touching highly erotic as the skin becomes suffused with sensual feelings. If you are applying the oils from Recipe 1, the basil essence will increase her responses to sensual touch, while the lavender and patchouli will soothe her skin. In Recipe 2, the aphrodisiac properties of neroli will complement its skin-nurturing qualities. Bergamot will entice her, while black pepper will warm and seduce her.

RECIPE 2

Tantalizing

Neroli, Bergamot,
Black Pepper

For all over skin
contact

To 4tsp base oil mix of the
above ingredients add:

4 drops Neroli
3 drops Bergamot
2 drops Black Pepper

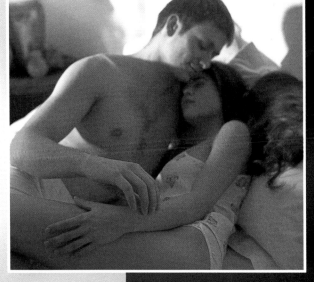

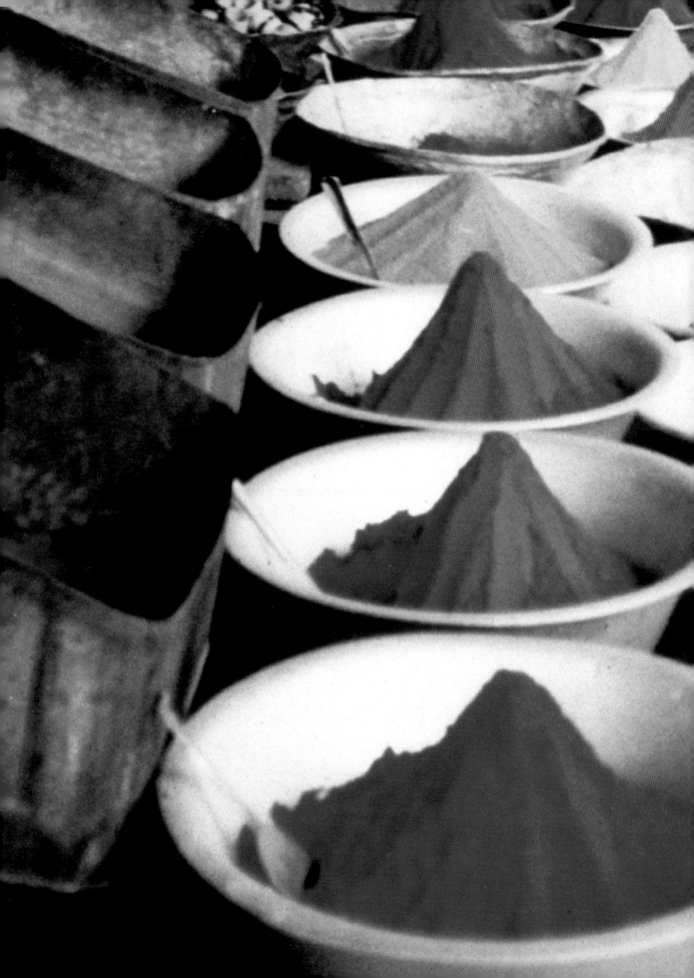

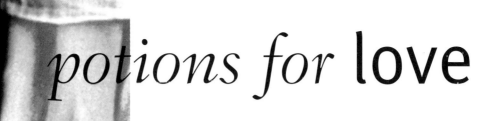

potions for love

CHAPTER 5 ▶

There is always a touch of magic in love and romance. It is as if something of the beyond enters us when we fall in love and lights up our lives so that even ordinary things become extraordinary. Love has the power, for a while at least, to dissolve our ego boundaries, opening us up to new and wonderful feelings and a sense of merging with the other. When we fall in love, our senses heighten, so that everything becomes brighter, more vivid and alive.

Love is an energy beyond our control, but it answers to an invitation. So when romance is in the air, take time to beckon it into your heart. This chapter shows you ways to use the gifts of nature for their healing and seductive properties and create your own love magic. It will inspire you to concoct your own love potions within the alluring backdrop of a beautifully prepared, sensual, and fragrant ambience (See Chapter 3). Prepare delicious meals for that special person, using the natural foods of love; feed each other exotic foods and toast each other's happiness from magical goblets filled with the juice of sexy fruits, wines, and spices. Use your essential oils, either as a balm to the body or in an aromatherapy burner, to release their fragrant invitation to love and romance. Let them ease away painful memories from the past, lifting the clouds from your heart so that you can embrace the new events in your life. Use the oils to welcome romance and to evoke the love spirits within yourself, increasing your potent sensual and sexual energies.

In a well-stocked kitchen, you can find all sorts of aphrodisiac aids, nestling innocently in the vegetable basket, the fruit bowl, and harboring in spice racks and herb jars. For nature has endowed many of her plants with amorous properties as well as the necessary nutrients for our basic sustenance. Many foods have long enjoyed the reputation of being erotic stimulants, and in the past were frequently used in potions and remedies to increase libido, induce fertility, or even to cast a seductive spell on the object of one's desire. Natural foods provide our bodies with essential nutrients, vitamins, minerals, essential fatty acids, amino acids, and carbohydrates. They give us the vitality and stamina to function, and that includes the energy to make love. Vegetables which are identified for their aphrodisiac qualities include: carrots, cucumbers, cress, onions, truffle mushrooms, asparagus, artichokes, radishes, celery, bamboo shoots, water chestnuts, tomatoes, and even the more mundane cabbages, parsnips, and potatoes.

Fruits, of course, with their succulent juices and sensual textures, and their prolific seeds, have always had a mythical association with sexuality and fecundity. Those which have erotic connotations include dates, figs, grapes, mangoes, pomegranates, peaches, bananas, persimmon, litchis, strawberries, avocados, guavas, and passion fruit. In Celtic and Greek mythology, nuts are synonymous with the quality of wisdom, but are also associated with love and sexuality. Pine nuts, pistachios, filberts, coconuts, chestnuts, walnuts, and almonds have all gained their aphrodisiac credentials throughout the centuries.

Herbs and spices, probably because of their warming and stimulating properties, were once greatly feared and condemned by puritans for being altogether too sexy and a threat to virtue. Garlic, for instance, has always enjoyed a fine reputation as an aid to virility and sexual stamina. Topping the list of aphrodisiac herbs and spices to add flavor and zest to your food are cinnamon, basil, pepper, cardamon, cloves, chilies, ginger, rosemary, vanilla, saffron, fennel, nutmeg, mint, sage, thyme, and cayenne.

So with all these evocative foods in mind, time spent in the kitchen should be less of a chore and more of a sensual experience. To make it more so, you can arrange the fruits, vegetables, nuts, and legumes, to make the most of their rich array of earthy colors and erotic shapes. Enjoy the wonderful mouthwatering aromas of fresh herbs and spices, especially when ground in a mortar and pestle. You can also use the essential oil recipes suggested here in an aromatherapy burner to harmonize your kitchen smells. Essence of bergamot with its sweet, refreshing perfume will stimulate your appetite as you cook and dispel overpowering odors such as garlic and onions. Or use the second recipe to combine rosemary, thyme, and lavender oils to purify the air while instilling into your kitchen the fragrance of an herbaceous country garden.

FOODS OF LOVE

RECIPE 1

Stimulating the

Appetite

Bergamot

To an aromatherapy burner

add the following

essential oil:

5 drops of Bergamot

RECIPE 2

Country Garden

Smells

Thyme, Rosemary and

Lavender

To an aromatherapy burner

add the following

essential oils:

2 drops Thyme

3 drops Rosemary

3 drops Lavender

SETTING A TABLE FOR LOVE

SETTING A TABLE FOR LOVE

RECIPE 1

Romance

Bergamot, Ginger, Lavender
To an aromatherapy burner
add the following
essential oils:
3 drops Bergamot
2 drops Ginger
3 drops Lavender

RECIPE 2

Seduction

Jasmine, Black Pepper,
Orange
To an aromatherapy burner
add the following
essential oils:
2 drops Jasmine
3 drops Black Pepper
3 drops Orange

While we may have lost much of our inherent knowledge about the amorous nature of food, many a love liaison is still forged over a romantic dinner for two. A carefully prepared meal in an ambient setting is as capable of working its magic now as it was in the past. Food and sex have been forever intertwined. We say we are "hungry for love" or we have an "appetite for sex". We talk about adding "spice" to our love-lives, or describe a particularly licentious affair as "juicy" or "fruity."

Weave magic into your relationship by preparing your loved one a special meal. Create a certain ambience to enhance the mood of your desire. If it is to be a purely romantic occasion, then use delicate colors to grace the table and inspire a soft and gentle feeling. Add a vase of honeysuckle, apple blossom, daisies, or freesias, or place a glass or ceramic bowl of water in the center of the table, scattering apple or orange blossom or rose petals into it to float on top. Light candles which are blue or pink to inspire the love, and in the background, play soft, sweet music. For a romantic dinner, perfume the room by adding drops of bergamot, ginger, and lavender essential oils to an aromatherapy burner (see Recipe 1) and create a fragrance that is uplifting and warm, yet is still soothing and relaxing.

If, however, your meal is intended to be provocative prelude to a sexy encounter, then surround yourself with deep, rich hues of red and burgundy, for the colors of red vibrate with and awaken the body's sex center. Use candlelight, or switch on a lamp which casts a warm and seductive glow in the room. Scatter soft-to-the-touch rose petals over the tablecloth, or add a vase of mixed red and cream tulips, selecting those which are just beginning to open out their petals sensuously. Select earthy, erotic background music and light an aromatherapy burner with the ingredients of Recipe 2, so that the jasmine, black pepper, and orange fragrances infuse the air with their warmth and spice to kindle the flame of passion.

PREPARE A SALAD OF EXOTIC

FRUITS TO FEED EACH OTHER.

You may like to prepare a meal of varying courses, or make a picnic of delicious tidbits. Choose your cuisine from the aphrodisiac foods listed on the previous page, adding to them any ingredients that you know your partner especially enjoys. Whatever your choice of food, combine their colors to look appealing, for a plate of insipid-looking food will inspire neither love nor lust. Remember that red is a sexually provocative color, while green is warming to the heart. Select different textures of food, first crisp and crunchy and then soft and succulent. Never overload the plates with food, but savor each deli-

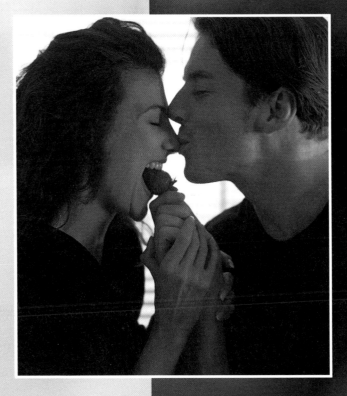

cious morsel for its own sensual flavor and taste. Enjoy the full vitality of natural foods to make the most of their aphrodisiac properties, so make sure to include them in a fresh green salad.

A DRINK
TO HEALTH AND
HAPPINESS

In almost every culture in the world, there is a common ritual where people raise their glasses and drink to health and happiness. Usually each country has a special salutation, among others, it could be "cheers," "juste," "schol," or "salute." More often than not, someone will pronounce a specific wish for good luck to one or all. In a sense, this is a moment of magical intent created within a circle of friends, for although it may be a common practice, it symbolizes a commu-

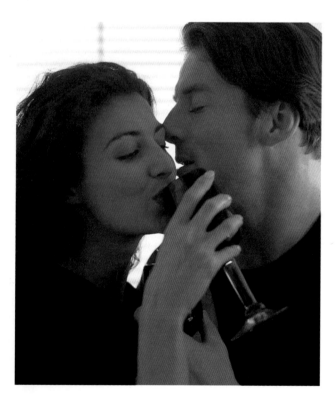

nal invocation to the positive forces of life. To wish someone health and happiness is to want the best for them.

When a couple raise their glasses to each other, they too are creating a magic spell – for even while they salute each other's health, they are also calling up the spirit of love. Lifting the glasses, their eyes will meet and they may say: "Here's to us," and in that moment of intimate contact, they are creating or affirming their mutual bond.

Turn your toast to love, health, and happiness into a special ritual for you and your partner. Prepare the drinks with care,

RAISE YOUR GOBLET AND DRINK

TO THE SPIRIT OF LOVE

pouring them into beautiful receptacles saved only for these occasions. Goblets are a perfect choice, their deep bowls and long stems evoking an erotic image of the molding of male and female sexuality. They are the cups associated with a bygone age, adding a little romance and mystery to a lover's brew. Or use cut crystal glasses for their pristine purity and their touch of luxury. Sparkling champagne or a good wine is the natural choice for many people who wish to propose a romantic toast. Alcohol, when taken in small quantities, is a well-known aphrodisiac, for it eases tension, reduces inhibitions, and can lighten the spirit, but care must be taken for an excess of alcohol can dampen any libido.

If alcohol is not desired, then you can make an elixir of exotic fruits. Select from the list of aphrodisiac fruits on page 94. Have fun in preparing your fruity love drink, picking your ingredients carefully for their erotic properties. For example, in classical mythology, fresh figs represent phallic virility, while the purple grape symbolizes the juice of life and sexual excess; apricots, peaches, and pears embody the essence of female sensuality. Blend your chosen fruits into a liquid pulp and slowly sup the potent juices together. Or, on a summer's night, make a creamy milkshake, blending your fruit together with three-quarters of a cup of milk, two scoops of vanilla ice cream, a few drops of vanilla extract and a sprinkle of ground cinnamon and nutmeg. The vanilla, cinnamon, and nutmeg will all add their aphrodisiac magic to the delicious cocktail.

Light a scent burner to enhance the mood of your toast to health, happiness, and love. The aroma of lavender will contribute to emotional harmony and stimulate the body's natural resources, lime will add a playful, party spirit and patchouli will deepen the sense of the wild and exotic.

A DRINK TO HEALTH AND HAPPINESS

RECIPE 1

Love, Health and Happiness

Lavender, Lime, Patchouli

To an aromatherapy burner add the following essential oils:

3 drops Lavender

2 drops Lime

1 drop Patchouli

INVOKING THE GOD AND GODDESS WITHIN

INVOKING THE GOD AND GODDESS WITHIN

Recipes for the Goddesses

RECIPE 1
Demeter/Wisdom
Frankincense
Add 3 drops of Frankincense to 1tsp jojoba oil and apply to the forehead.

RECIPE 2
Venus/Love
Rose
Add 3 drops of Rose to 1tsp jojoba oil and apply to the heart area.

RECIPE 3
Aphrodite/Sensuality/ Sexuality
Ylang Ylang
Add 3 drops of Ylang Ylang to 1tsp jojoba oil and apply to the abdomen.

In classical mythology, tales of the gods and goddesses, satyrs, nymphs, and woodland sprites are bound completely with a love and respect of nature and the verdant vegetation of the ancient sun-drenched Mediterranean land.

Many of these deities were associated not only with certain trees, flowers, or herbs, but also with specific qualities, such as the spirit of wisdom, love, or sensuality. The gods and goddesses of the Greek and Roman pantheon, although portrayed as immortals, can be viewed, in fact, as archetypes of particular characteristics which are important to us all.

Whenever you feel something is missing from your life, take the time to playfully invoke the relevant spirit of the gods and goddesses. The ceremony, using a selection of the essential oils recommended on this page, will help to return the feeling of abundance back into your relationship. What you are doing, in fact, is simply opening yourself up to the rich and diverse nature of your own psyche. The aroma of each of the

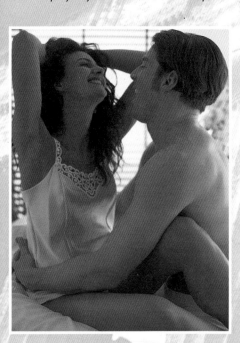

RECAPTURE THE SPIRIT OF PLAYFULNESS

chosen oils will resonate with the particular character and spirit of your chosen deity when applied to a relevant part of your body. Each of these areas is connected to a specific energy center or *chakra* corresponding to the essence of love, sensuality, and wisdom.

If you are a woman, choose frankincense oil to invoke the spirit of Demeter, goddess of wisdom and mental order; rose to call up Venus, who represents the heart and the power of love; or ylang ylang to summon up the sensuality and sexuality of Aphrodite. For a man, select cedarwood to encourage the wisdom and clarity of Apollo; sandalwood for the physical sensuality and ecstatic love nature of Dionysius; or patchouli for the musky, earthy sexuality of Pan.

You may be aware of what is missing in your life, or you can conduct a simple ceremony, either alone or with your lover, to ascertain which of these energies you need to enhance. Sit silently in a warm and peaceful room, lit only by the flames of a fire or some pure white candles. Place bowls of potpourri around the room to create the spirit of the woodlands and meadows. Breathe deeply and begin to relax your body and mind. After some minutes, place both hands, one on top of the other, softly over your lower abdomen for up to two minutes and focus your breath and attention into this area. Then repeat this procedure on the solar plexus area, heart, and forehead. If any of these areas feel cold or less vibrant than other areas, you may sense which deity or spirit you need to evoke. Rub the appropriate oil into that part of your body to recapture the playful spirit of one of nature's gods.

INVOKING THE GOD AND GODDESS WITHIN

Recipes for the Gods

RECIPE 1

Apollo/Wisdom

Cedarwood

Add 3 drops of Cedarwood to 1tsp jojoba oil and apply to the forehead.

RECIPE 2

Dionysius/ Ecstatic Love

Sandalwood

Add 3 drops of Sandalwood to 1tsp jojoba oil and apply to the solar plexus and heart areas.

RECIPE 3

Pan/ Earthy Sexuality

Patchouli

Add 3 drops of Patchouli to 1tsp jojoba oil and apply to the abdomen.

HEALING
THE HEART

RECIPES FOR HEALING THE HEART

Choose 2 or 3 oils from an appropriate category of Emotionally Healing Oils listed on the opposite page

RECIPE 1

Aromatherapy burner
or Bath

To an aromatherapy burner or bath add the following:

7 drops of an oil blended from up to 3 essential oils from your chosen category.

RECIPE 2

Anointing Yourself

To every 4tsp of unperfumed moisturiser add the following:

6 drops of oil blended from up to 3 essential oils from any chosen category.

Just as new love brings in its wake feelings of renewed hope and happiness, so too does the end of a love relationship carry its own energy of hurt, pain, and sadness. Most people have known the experience of a broken heart, when it seems as if the heart has splintered into a thousand fragments, turning positive emotions into those of bitter disillusionment. This is a devastating period for anyone to go through, for it can leave us racked with insecurity, painful emotions, and obsessive thoughts.

So it is important to allow time for inner healing as the emotional wounds need to be felt and faced up to, in order to let them go. If not, they can bury themselves deep into the psyche and act subconsciously on our self-esteem and confidence, setting up patterns of behavior which can harm the potential of a new relationship.

Nature's essential oils can play a very healing role at a time like this, for their soothing properties and aromas have a direct effect on our emotional responses, affecting the limbic part of the brain that controls memory and emotion. So take good care of yourself, and immerse yourself in every possible way with these supportive, nurturing oils, selecting them as appropriate from the lists given below. For 2 to 3 days, have a fragrant feast. Burn the oils in your scent burner around the house, especially in the bedroom, to banish your environment of old and painful memories. Treat yourself to a whole-body massage, for you deserve to be pampered, and have the essential oils recommended here added to the massage oil blend. Bathe yourself in the steaming aroma of the oils, luxuriating in their calming, cleansing properties, then add them to an unperfumed lotion to spread onto your skin so their benefits seep into every pore. Create your own perfumes by mixing the essences into a base oil, and dab it onto your wrists and behind your ears, or onto your temples so that you carry the fragrance with you wherever you go.

Give yourself time to allow the feelings of hurt to arise, and when you have fully accepted them, banish them from your heart. Be positive and tell yourself that this will pass. Willingly let go of old and familiar memories and then look ahead with excitement to the new and unknown.

The following list are the essential oils you can use to heal the heart. Select one or three oils from the appropriate categories which relate to your pain or needs and blend them according to the recipes given on this page.

Communication of difficult issues: clary sage, ylang ylang, geranium, frankincense, lavender.

Rejection: juniper, lavender, patchouli, rose, bergamot, geranium, jasmine.

Jealousy: Rose, ylang ylang.

Infidelity: juniper, sandalwood.

Breach of trust: juniper, frankincense, jasmine.

Grief: rose, neroli, cedarwood.

Healing painful emotions: rose, black pepper, sandalwood, ginger.

RECIPE 3

For Massage

To a 5tsp base oil mix of jojoba, sweet almond and avocado add the following: *14 drops of oil blended from up to 3 essential oils from any chosen category.*

LET THE OILS HELP TO HEAL

A BROKEN HEART

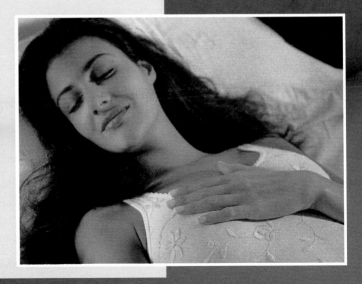

INVITING A
NEW ROMANCE

INVITING A
NEW ROMANCE

Recipes for Courage

RECIPE 1

Cedarwood, Sandalwood,
Basil, Geranium
To Aromatherapy burner or
bath add the following:
5 drops of a combination of
the above essential oils

RECIPE 2

Anointing Yourself

Cedarwood, Sandalwood,
Basil, Ginger
To 4tsp base of jojoba oil
add the following:
6 drops of a combination of 3
of the above essential oils

Before you are ready to open yourself up to a new romance, you may first need to give yourself courage, and for this reason, you can anoint yourself, bathe in or place in an aromatherapy burner one or two of the following oils: cedarwood, sandalwood, basil, or ginger. (See Recipe 1 & 2). Then, whenever you are ready, you can use your essential oils to invite a happy relationship back into your life.

The following visualization technique, together with the magic of your essential oils, will allow you to draw consciously to yourself the kind of person you want to attract by encapturing the spirit of your ideal man or woman. To do this, you need first to choose or create a seductive environment in which to visualize exactly what you are looking for in a romance. Place lighted blue candles in all four corners of your bathroom, and soak yourself in a warm and steaming bath or sit meditatively before the flickering flames of a fire. Use an aromatherapy burner to fill the air with the beautiful scent of rose and cedarwood to open the heart and con-

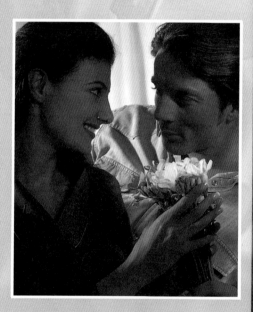

THE AROMATIC OILS CAN HELP YOU TO OPEN UP TO LOVE

CHARACTER OILS

BASIL: *strong and assertive*

BERGAMOT: *content and devoted*

BLACK PEPPER: *warm and loving*

CEDARWOOD: *calm and focused*

CLARY SAGE: *wild and passionate*

FRANKINCENSE: *spiritual and communicative*

GERANIUM: *energetic and well-balanced*

GINGER: *passionate and motivated*

JASMINE: *achiever and confident*

LAVENDER: *even-tempered and nurturing*

LIME: *playful and charming*

NEROLI: *relaxed and imaginative*

ORANGE: *funny and youthful*

PATCHOULI: *earthy and faithful*

ROSE: *gentle and with integrity*

SANDALWOOD: *intellectual and sensual*

YLANG YLANG: *romantic and innocent*

centrate the mind and spirit (see Recipe for Visualization). Or go outside into the backyard, forest or meadow, and sit beside a cedar or another evergreen tree or a beautiful rose bush. Relax and breathe deeply so you attain a sense of inner equilibrium. Now allow your thoughts to form a gradual image of the person you desire. What are his or her main characteristics? Do you want an honest, practical earthy type, or a more spiritual and intellectual person. Try to envision at least 2 to 3 of the most important characterists that you would seek in a lover. Tell yourself you are worthy of attracting these qualities and that you deserve a lasting happiness. Once you have attained a rounded picture of your ideal partner, take the time to write their attributes down on paper.

Now look through the above list for the character types and the corresponding essential oil. Mix together a blend of the most appropriate oils into a base oil of jojoba. (See Recipes for Character Oils). Wear this blend daily, remembering to visualize the person of your dreams whenever you anoint your body. Once you meet your new romance, your perfume will bind that person to you, for you have already captured his or her heart and spirit.

Recipe for Visualization

Cedarwood, Rose

To an aromatherapy burner add the following:

4 drops Cedarwood

3 drops Rose

Recipe for the Ideal Lover

See Character Oils listed on this page

To 4tsp jojoba oil base add the following:

6 drops of a combination of 2 to 3 Character Essential Oils blended to the appropriate strengths of preference.

HEALING
SEXUAL TENSION
Men

HEALING SEXUAL TENSION

Recipes for Men

RECIPE 1

Sexual Anxiety

*Clary Sage, Jasmine,
Patchouli*

To an aromatherapy burner
add the following:

4 drops Jasmine

1 drop Clary Sage

1 drop Patchouli

For massage:

To 5tsp base oil mix of above
ingredients add:

7 drops Jasmine

3 drops Patchouli

3 drops Clary Sage

RECIPE 2

Sexual Dysfunction

Jasmine, Sandalwood

To an aromatherapy burner
add the following:

3 drops Jasmine

2 drops Sandalwood

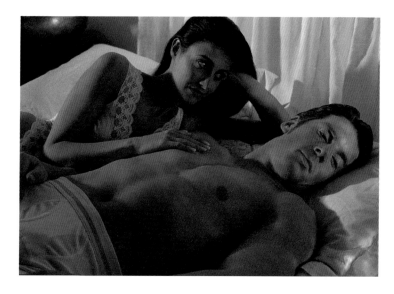

THE AROMATIC OILS WILL HELP TO SOOTHE HIS SEXUAL TENSION

Essential oils can be very beneficial in easing sexual anxiety, soothing fears that may stand in the way of the full enjoyment of an intimate relationship. Certain aromas exact their influence on the olfactory senses, stimulating the body, relaxing the mind, opening the heart, and warming the emotions. They can help draw you away from far distant thoughts and distractions into the sensual experience of the present moment.

Everyone goes through periods when the libido is low. This may be the result of stress, either at home or in work, when it seems impossible to free your mind from a web of worries. Serious stress can have a marked effect on your interest in sex, for it causes you to withdraw from your body and to contract emotionally. If you are locked in problems, it seems hardly possible to surrender to the sensations of body pleasure. Or, if you are angry with your partner, and a situation remains unresolved, then it may not be possible to suddenly switch yourself back to warm and loving feelings. These are the times when understanding and support from your partner can help you to resolve your tensions. The aromatic oils will assist you, and if you study their profiles (see Chapter 1), you can become familiar with their particular aphrodisiac or emotionally evocative properties. Try to understand exactly what is disturbing you and where your needs lie, so that you can carefully choose specific oils to enhance the sensuality of your body, soothe your mind, or raise your spirit – or oils which bring a balance between all three. You can follow the recipes shown here or on the following page, which have been chosen especially for their enhancing effects on male and female sexual issues.

If you are a man and you are hoping to make love for the first time to a new partner, or if you have not made love for a long time, you may be anxious about the event. Take things slowly until you feel comfortable with your new partner, letting your sexual relationship unfold like a flower. If you have the opportunity, place a scent burner in your bedroom – your lover will appreciate its perfume (Recipe 1). If the problems are more long-term, then ask an understanding partner to massage you regularly with the essential oils (Recipe 2). It may be necessary to seek professional help with your sexual problems, but the aromatic massage will help relax your body and ease sexual tensions while soothing your mind. Her touch will nurture you, helping you regain your self esteem.

For massage:
To 5tsp base oil mix of sweet almond and grapeseed add the following:
6 drops Jasmine
5 drops Sandalwood

RECIPE 3
Raising Libido
Black Pepper, Ginger, Sandalwood
To an aromatherapy burner add the following:
2 drops Black Pepper
3 drops Ginger
2 drops Sandalwood
For massage:
To base oil mix of above mentioned ingredients add the following:
3 drops Ginger,
3 drops Black Pepper
6 drops Sandalwood

HEALING
SEXUAL TENSION
Women

HEALING SEXUAL TENSION

RECIPE 1

Sexual Anxiety

Jasmine, Sandalwood, Neroli

To an aromatherapy burner

add the following:

2 drops Jasmine

2 drops Sandalwood

3 drops Neroli

For Massage:

To 4tsp base oil mix of

sweet almond and grapeseed

add the following:

3 drops Jasmine

4 drops Sandalwood

4 drops Neroli

RECIPE 2

Sexual Dysfunction

Rose, Ylang Ylang

To an aromatherapy burner

add the following:

4 drops Rose

3 drops Ylang Ylang

Aromatic oils are equally effective on women in helping them to feel more comfortable in a sexual situation. If you are nervous about making love, either because you are just entering into an intimate relationship, or you have not made love for a long time, then surround yourself with healing fragrances which will soothe away your fears. Place jasmine, sandalwood, and neroli in a scent burner so its perfume fills your bedroom, and breathe deeply to inhale the smell of this wonderful and exotically sensual blend. Jasmine and sandalwood will help you to feel as if you are really back inside your body instead of being locked up with your mind. Neroli will enhance the blend, surrounding you with the haunting fragrance used and loved by Cleopatra. Neroli is a particularly appropriate choice of oil in times of sexual anxiety, for it is both a relaxant and an aphrodisiac. It is able to combine a deep and soothing feeling of peace and contentment while putting you in the mood for love. It will also give you the courage to communicate about your sexual fears or any issues of importance which exist between you and your lover. This communication will enable your relationship to go deeper.

If you feel that you have a sexual dysfunction, then seek professional help from a counsellor or doctor, for it may have a medical base. Or it may be rooted in painful memories or emotional issues, which an expert sex therapist can help you to resolve. At the same time, use the rose and ylang ylang oils to heal past emotional wounds and to awaken your innate sensuality. Anoint yourself with the luxuriant blends, and enjoy touching your own body. Nurture your

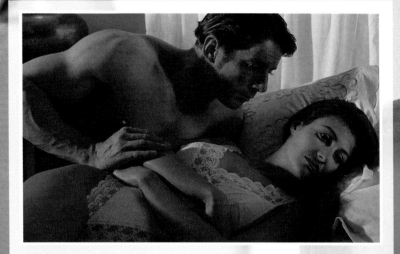

ALLOW STRESS TO DISSOLVE UNDER THE INFLUENCE OF THE OILS

skin as you stroke and caress yourself. Have a friend or lover massage you with these oils, and enjoy the experience of being pampered (Recipe 1). Essence of rose will make you feel enticing, seductive, and exquisitely feminine. This flower of Venus will heal your heart, opening it up to gentle and loving feelings. If you are nervous, it will calm you and create positive thoughts in your mind. Combine your rose oil with ylang ylang oil, for it too can open up your heart to love and your body to sensuality. It can also ease old feelings of guilt or worry which may inhibit your free-flowing sexual energy.

Perhaps you are simply tired or lethargic, or stress has lowered your vitality and caused you to lose interest in sex. Choose oils which will warm you up (Recipe 2). Black pepper and ginger should do the trick, putting the spice back into your life. Then add a little neroli for a really seductive and sensuous feel. Place your oils in a burner or ask your friend to give you a lovely massage.

For massage:
To 4tsp base of above
mentioned ingredients add
the following:
5 drops Rose
4 drops Ylang Ylang

RECIPE 3
Increasing Libido
Black Pepper, Ginger, Neroli
To an aromatherapy burner
add the following:
2 drops Black Pepper
2 drops Ginger
3 drops Neroli

For massage:
To 4tsp base oil mix of above
mentioned ingredients add
the following:
4 drops Black Pepper
3 drops Ginger
4 drops Neroli

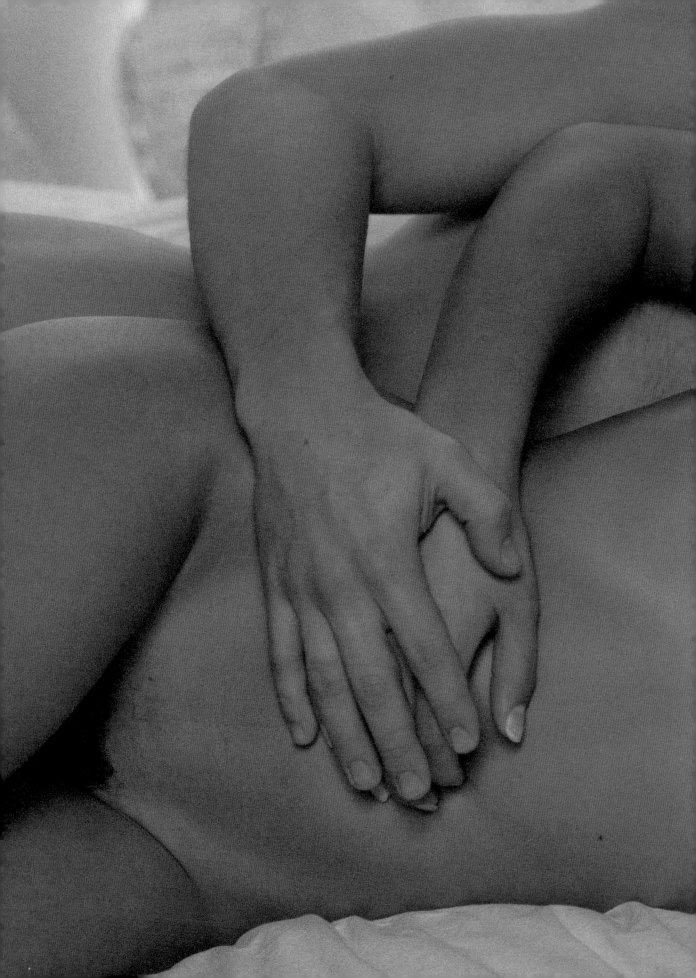

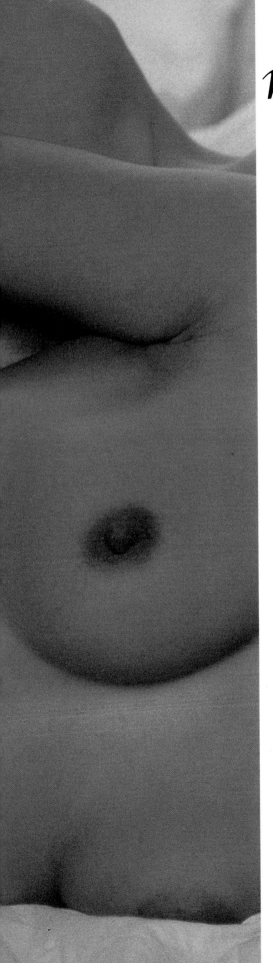

making love

Holistic sexuality involves the body, mind, and spirit and makes no division between them. It is an invitation for the two people concerned to bring themselves physically, emotionally, and spiritually into the act of making love. This requires finding a deep level of honesty, trust, and intimacy within yourself and then sharing this naked vulnerability with your lover. If you and your partner are willing to take this journey together, then making love can become an art and a ritual of the highest form. Sensual aromatherapy can enhance this mutual experience. The fragrant oils, blended to your personal choice or appropriate recipes, will infuse the sensual ambience you have prepared with their nature-given properties. Some of the oils will help you grow in trust, soothing away the hurts and wounds of the past which have kept your heart defended against the pure and poignant arrow of love. Other aromas will warm the emotions and uplift the spirit, bringing playfulness and joy to the moment. Choose and select your oils to aid sexual healing, or to act as an aphrodisiac to heighten your sexual responses. When the oils act their magic, the two of you can explore the internal and external world of senses, feelings, and essential energy. Celebrate special memories and surrender to the awakening power of your sexuality, letting it take you, like a river merging into the ocean, into something greater and beyond yourselves.

AWAKENING THE SENSES

AWAKENING THE SENSES

RECIPE 1

Expanding

Basil, Frankincense, Lavender

To an aromatherapy burner

add the following:

1 drop Basil

2 drops Frankincense

3 drops Lavender

RECIPE 2

Focusing

Cedarwood, Black Pepper,

Bergamot

To an aromatherapy burner

add the following:

4 drops Cedarwood

5 drops Black Pepper

6 drops Bergamot

Sight, sound, smell, taste, and touch are the five senses of the body through which we define our experiences of life. When our senses are heightened, we feel alive and vibrant and connected from the depth of our being to the world beyond. The physical senses touch and effect every aspect of our mental, emotional, and spiritual make-up. The sight of a beautiful flower, the song of a bird, the perfume of a rose, the satisfaction of good food, and the caress of a lover can fill us with happiness, affect our thoughts positively, and uplift our spirit.

While we need and use all of our senses in everyday life, we tend to neglect their full potential. Stress and concern can dull our senses, narrowing them down to a purely functional level. Yet we are sentient beings with a huge capacity to experience pleasure through

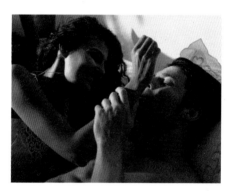

BREATHE IN THE AROMA OF THE ESSENTIAL OIL BLEND SHE HAS PLACED ON HER WRIST

the body. Taking the time to awaken them will heighten our enjoyment of life. Love is one of the energies which expands our senses and heightens our perceptions. When we first fall in love, colors become more vivid, smells more intense, sounds more vibrant, taste more delicious, and touch more exquisite. The world, with its sky and stars, trees and flowers, birds and people suddenly becomes a wonderful place. Recapture those heightened senses with the use of your essential oils and play a sensory awareness exercise with your partner. Choose either shown here for a sensory-enhancing blend.

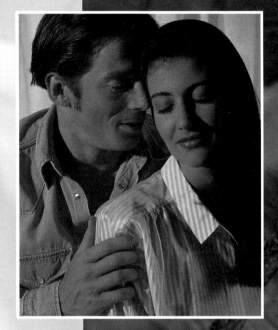

Do the exercise in turn. If you are the passive partner sit quietly, spending a few moments letting go of thoughts and concerns. Wait for your partner to surprise and awaken each of your senses. Focus all of your attention on the immediate sensation before you. If he gives you a flower, take time to absorb the beauty of its shape and color. Then touch each petal to feel its silky texture. Lift it to your nose to breathe in its perfume. If he plays some music for you, chimes resonate bells, or whispers into your ear, let your hearing expand to capture all the nuances of sound. He can then stimulate your taste buds, putting into your mouth, one piece at a time, some tiny morsels of delicious food. Close your eyes and concentrate completely on savoring each specific taste and texture. Then he can draw your attention to your tactile sense. Feel your skin tingle in response to every teasing stimulation. He can stroke his fingertips lightly over your skin, or trail soft textures of silk and chiffon against your face – notice the varying sensations on the different parts of your body and what feels warm or cool on your skin. Lose yourself completely in every sensation until all of your senses have become totally awakened.

WHISPER SWEET WORDS IN HER EAR

MEDITATION FOR LOVE

MEDITATING TOGETHER

RECIPE 1

Meditation

Frankincense, Sandalwood

To an aromatherapy burner

add the following:

4 drops Frankincense

3 drops Sandalwood

RECIPE 2

Love and Devotion

Rose, Cedarwood, Clary Sage

To an aromatherapy burner

add the following:

2 drops Rose

2 drops Cedarwood

2 drops Clary Sage

Meditating with your partner can enhance the feeling of peace and harmony within your relationship and open your hearts to the essential energy of love. When practiced regularly, even for a short period each day, it can calm the mind in times of turmoil and stress.

To enhance your meditation, create an environment which helps you to sit silently and focus on your breathing. Choose a quiet place in your home, and light a candle and then surround yourself with the aroma of frankincense and sandalwood. Both oils will enhance the mood of meditation and contemplation, encouraging your hearts to open without reservation. They are the oils used in places of worship throughout the world to inspire devotion. Frankincense expands and elevates the spirit, while sandalwood awakens the physical senses. Both help you to relax into the present moment of reality in body, mind, and soul. Place your oils in an aromatherapy burner to infuse the air with their woody and inspiring fragrance.

One of the main techniques of meditation is the awareness of breath, because breathing is our fundamental link to life, and the connection between our inner and outer worlds. Breath is the source of our vitality. When our breath is relaxed and deep, it washes through every cell of the body, relaxes the mind, and expands our consciousness. Frankincense helps to open and deepen the breathing and expand the lungs, thus making us feel more alive and at the same time more calm.

Sitting together in your candle-lit room, for a period of between 15 to 40 minutes, close your eyes and begin to focus your attention on your breath. Do not try to change it in any way, just be aware of it moving in and out through your body. Whenever you become distracted by your thoughts, focus back on your breathing. You cannot stop the thoughts in your mind but gradually you can become less involved in them. Breath awareness will draw you away from your restless mind towards a more silent place within.

After you have sat together in this way for a number of occasions, and you feel relaxed with the breathing meditation, you may like to do a special ritual dedicated to the energy of love.

Use rose, cedarwood, and clary sage essential oils in your burner, for their properties will combine to expand your feelings of love, devotion, and surrender toward each other. Sit facing each other and take each other's hands, pouring yourself into this connection as if the two of you were united in body, mind, and spirit. Focus your attention onto your heart *chakra*, and as you exhale, imagine that you are softly breathing out all the love you have inside to let it embrace your lover. Then breathe in as if you are absorbing your partner's love for you. Turn your cycle of breathing into a circle of love.

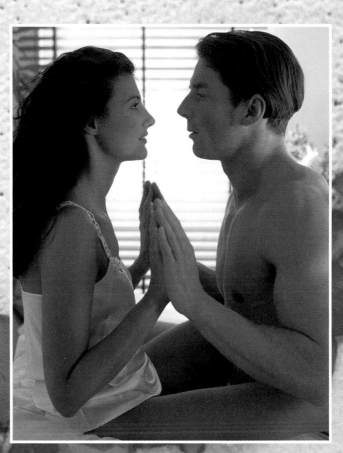

CREATE A CIRCLE OF LOVE BY HARMONIZING YOUR BREATHING TOGETHER

CELEBRATING THE BODY

CELEBRATING THE BODY

RECIPE 1

Celebrating Sexuality

Patchouli, Black Pepper,
Orange

To an aromatherapy burner

add the following:

2 drops Patchouli

3 drops Black Pepper

2 drops Orange

RECIPE 2

Celebrating Sensuality

Ylang Ylang, Black Pepper,
Patchouli

To an aromatherapy burner

add the following:

3 drops Ylang Ylang

3 drops Black Pepper

1 drop Patchouli

Our bodies can be a source of a great joy, but sometimes we carry fears and inhibitions which prohibit us from fully letting go into our potential of ecstasy. Those tensions may lock themselves in the body's muscles as well as burying themselves deep into the mind. Moving the body and letting it have free expression can dissolve the tensions that inhibits our more playful and spontaneous spirit.

Dancing to music can help us to free ourselves both physically and emotionally. It is one of the most powerful mediums of celebration known to men and women. Rhythm and sound can evoke the sensuality of the body, the emotions of love, and the feeling of spiritual awakening. All of these feelings can be manifested through physical movement; the stamping of feet and gyrating of the pelvis; the swaying of the body with arms uplifted as the heart is stirred and the gentle, almost imperceptible motion which moves through the body like a quiet breeze when the mind is lulled and the soul is uplifted. Celebrate your body and its vitality together with your partner. Choose aromatic oils which will encourage each aspect of your nature to express itself through your movements. Choose your music carefully, so that at one time you can be totally in the physical sensations of your body, and another time in the expression of your feelings, so that together you dance your love for each other. Clear your perfumed room so that you have the space to abandon yourself completely into movement. Remove your clothes so that you are naked and free, or leave on only those items which do not restrict you. Let go of your inhibitions and begin to dance, sometimes alone and sometimes together as the mood takes you. Find your own celebrative creativity and then let it harmonise with your lover's movements, so that it becomes one dance.

If you are dancing the dance of the wild, become free like a spirit of nature. Let your bodies go, stamping your feet and swaying your pelvis. Dance to the rhythm of the music and the perfumes of patchouli, black pepper, and orange, letting their earthy, warm, and sunshine energies stir your passions.

On another occasion, choose softer and more melodious music to express the more sensual and softer side of your nature. Be aware of the movements in your feet, legs, and pelvis, but focus more on your upper body, especially on the abdomen and chest, and let your arms open wide as your heart expands.

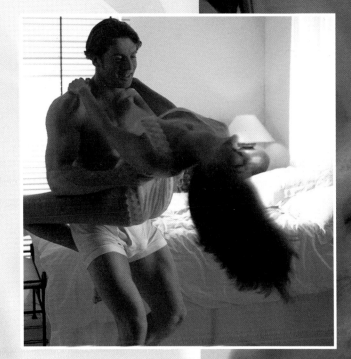

ABANDON YOURSELVES TO DANCE ENHANCED BY EROTIC SCENTS

Breathe deeply as you move, letting your bodies synchronize their movement. To encourage your sensual, loving feelings, add sweet, heady ylang ylang to a blend of patchouli and black pepper (see Recipe 2) and put it in your scent burner.

CELEBRATING
LOVE

Some days in the year hold special memories for a couple. It may be a birthday, Valentine's Day, or the anniversary of the day you met or married. Celebrate these days as a tribute to romance. By taking the time and trouble to create a special event, you are showing each other that you do not take your relationship for granted.

If you have the day free, spend it walking in the countryside or wood, letting the smells and sights of nature inspire and rejuvenate you. At home, or if you have had to spend the day at work, bathe together in a candle-lit bathroom, letting the fragrant oils seep into every pore of your skin. Infuse your home with the fragrance of romance by placing a blend of oils in your scent-burner. Recipe 1 shown here will enhance a deep sense of love and let-go. The clary sage will relax you deeply, helping you surrender to each euphoric moment. Rose will expand your feelings of love. Geranium will increase physical sensuality and give confidence and strength. Recipe 2 is for the spirit of fun if your mood is playful and sexy. The aroma of orange helps you to feel young and carefree and full of zest, while patchouli's perfume encourages your erotic and earthy sexuality. Frankincense will enhance and expand all of your senses so that every single stimulus can be fully enjoyed.

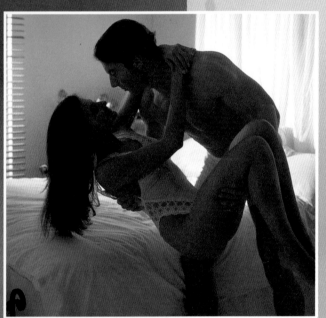

SWEEP HER INTO YOUR ARMS AND
CARRY HER INTO THE
FRAGRANCED BEDROOM

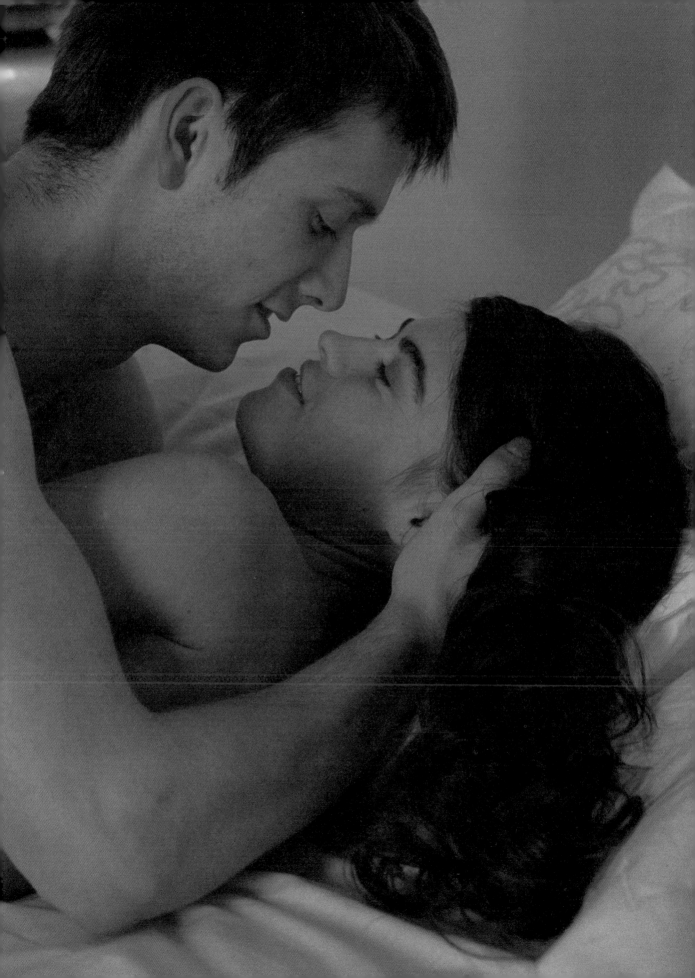

EROTIC TOUCHING

RECIPE 1

For the Man

Jasmine, Bergamot

To 5tsp base oil mix of jojoba
and sweet almond add the
following:

7 drops Jasmine

6 drops Bergamot

RECIPE 2

For the Woman

Neroli, Geranium

To 4tsp base oil mix of jojoba
and sweet almond add the
following:

7 drops Neroli

3 drops Geranium

Tactile contact is always a two-way sensation. You cannot touch the body of your lover without its touching you in return. Skin contact is where you both meet your lover and define yourself at the same time. As your hands caress her body, you feel its warmth and sensual softness. In the quality and care of your touch, she in turn experiences what you are feeling about her. As you stroke him, you express your attraction and love, and at the same time, you can sense whether he is responding and opening up to you. In fact, the moment you touch each other, two realities are meeting and merging.

Touch between lovers, whether it is in the context of massage (see Chapter 4, Therapeutic Massage) or part of their lovemaking, is a silent language through which you exchange deep communication. Verbally, you can say things without revealing your true emotions, but in the way you touch each other, you can never lie. Your touch on your lover's skin will speak directly to her heart, just as her skin responses will communicate her innermost feelings.

A loving touch during the time of foreplay and while making love should always honor the body of your partner. While stroking and caressing each other, try to remain in the present experience of sensation, rather than anticipating what will come next. Let every tender, erotic touch exist for its own sake and for the pleasure it brings rather than being a technique aimed at a pre-conceived goal. Let go of distracting thoughts and expectations, and pour yourself totally into your hands to stroke over the whole of your lover's body, enjoying the feel of the skin and its underlying structure. The human body is wonderfully sensual with its rounded shapes and curves. Do not rush, but let your hands linger lovingly to fully appreciate each part of it. Bring the whole of your consciousness into your touch and begin to imagine what it feels like to your partner's skin. Transport yourself into its very sensation, and as you do this, you will begin to feel as if the boundaries between your bodies are melting. Your touch and your lover's sensation begin to merge into one phenomenon, and even as you caress it will seem as if your partner is stroking you.

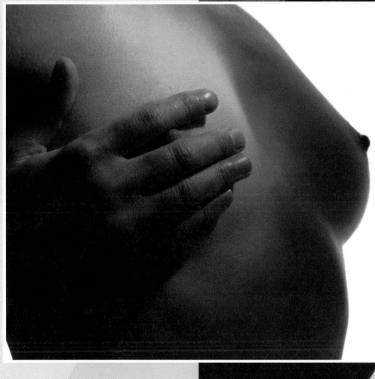

Erotic touching can be as nurturing as any other loving touch. However well you know each other, touch each other as if you were exploring the body for the first time. Let your touch convey wonder and respect. To make your erotic touching even more exotic, blend some essential oils into a mix of rich nutrient base oils such as jojoba and sweet almond, and apply to the skin. The woman can apply jasmine and bergamot to the man (Recipe 1), while neroli and geranium (Recipe 2) are the perfect blend for a woman's skin.

MAKING LOVE

RECIPES FOR MAKING LOVE

RECIPE 1

Playful Lovemaking

Lime, Ginger, Lavender

To an aromatherapy burner

add the following:

2 drops Lime

2 drops Lavender

3 drops Ginger

RECIPE 2

Gentle lovemaking

Frankincense, Ylang Ylang,

Bergamot

To an aromatherapy burner

add the following:

3 drops Frankincense

2 drops Ylang Ylang

2 drops Bergamot

Surround yourself with fragrance as you make love and let the character of the oils transport you and your partner into the realm of bliss. Now is the time for you to choose your own special blend, selecting those oils which have become significant to you and your partner, and with which you have developed a deep connection. Nobody else can really tell you what aroma will best suit your sexual encounters, for these moments are intensely personal to you both. The recipes recommended on these pages can be used as a guide, but it would be even better if you allowed your own sense of smell to direct you. Also, go back to the beginning of the book and look up the sensual and emotional properties of each oil, then try to tune in to what you need and what you are feeling, and let your intuition lead you. Involve your lover in this exploration so that you mutually find an aromatic blend which belongs just to the two of you. Wear this perfume on nights of love, or put it into the bedroom scent burner. If you massage each other before making love, you can also mix it into the base oil. You may even want to make a number of blends, which can reflect your changing moods. Store them in beautiful glass bottles so the oils are readily available if you wish to anoint each other.

Like the oils, making love will evoke and enhance your moods. It can bring you great happiness, it can make you laugh, and it can move you to tears. It can involve every emotion within you as you let go deeply into your feelings. It can awaken every sense in your body, taking you on a journey from sweet tenderness

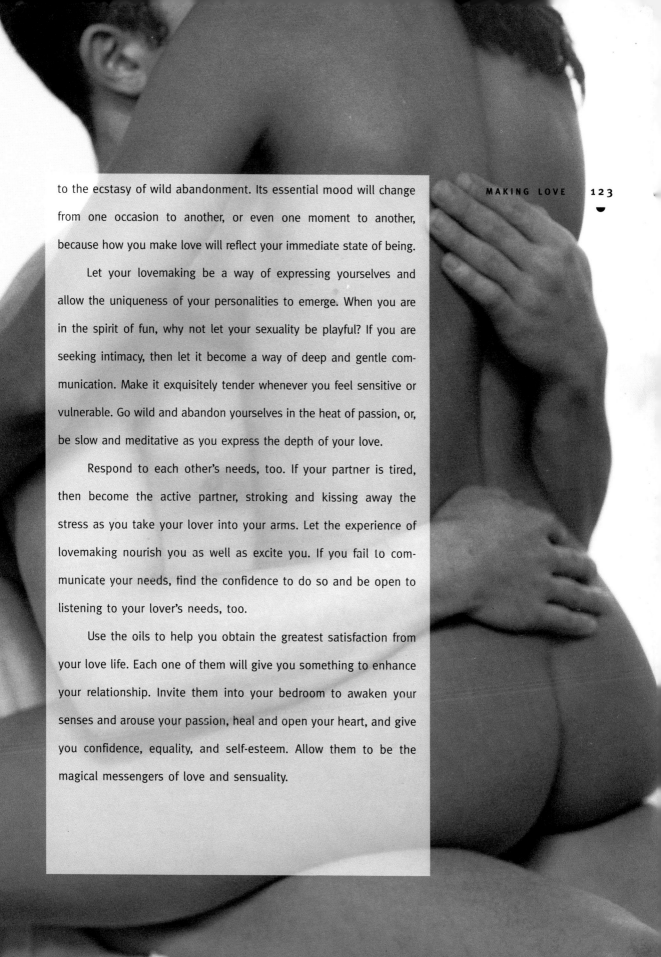

to the ecstasy of wild abandonment. Its essential mood will change from one occasion to another, or even one moment to another, because how you make love will reflect your immediate state of being.

Let your lovemaking be a way of expressing yourselves and allow the uniqueness of your personalities to emerge. When you are in the spirit of fun, why not let your sexuality be playful? If you are seeking intimacy, then let it become a way of deep and gentle communication. Make it exquisitely tender whenever you feel sensitive or vulnerable. Go wild and abandon yourselves in the heat of passion, or, be slow and meditative as you express the depth of your love.

Respond to each other's needs, too. If your partner is tired, then become the active partner, stroking and kissing away the stress as you take your lover into your arms. Let the experience of lovemaking nourish you as well as excite you. If you fail to communicate your needs, find the confidence to do so and be open to listening to your lover's needs, too.

Use the oils to help you obtain the greatest satisfaction from your love life. Each one of them will give you something to enhance your relationship. Invite them into your bedroom to awaken your senses and arouse your passion, heal and open your heart, and give you confidence, equality, and self-esteem. Allow them to be the magical messengers of love and sensuality.

MEDITATIVE SEXUALITY

Sexuality is a doorway to life's beautiful mysteries. It can answer our human needs and take us beyond them. The fusion of male and female energies in the context of love and awareness can become a transcendental experience. In this blissful experience lies sexuality's spiritual potential.

The belief that sexuality can transform consciousness has been honored in many traditions. It was known to the shamans of the Native Americans, and was central to the sacred rituals of the ancient Egyptians and Greeks. The Taoist teachers of China instructed their pupils carefully in the art of love, not only in pursuit of longevity, but also for spiritual reasons. Disciples of the Tantric teachings of India practiced sexo-yogic positions in pursuit of the state of enlightenment. In pagan and animist worship, people celebrated human sexuality as a tribute to the potency of nature. As more and more people these days seek to find more meaning in their lives and to enhance their state of well-being, so there has been a considerable revival in the concept of meditative sexuality.

If this is of interest to you and your partner, you can explore this dimension of sexuality within your relationship. Begin by meditating together regularly, using the oils suggested on pages 114-115 to enhance your inner feelings of peace. Learn to enjoy being with each other in this silent way. Massage each other regularly so your bodies become sensual and receptive and you become deeply in tune with each other.

When you are making love meditatively, you need to let go of thoughts and fantasies that take you away from the present moment. Focus completely on the here-and-now and each moment of being together. You will be making love in a cool way, rather than moving towards excitement and passion. When you feel yourselves becoming too aroused, slow down and breathe together. Try to keep your excitement level well below the threshold of orgasm, but let yourselves fully experience each sensation of breath and tactile contact. Stay deeply in tune with each other by breathing in harmony and making eye contact. Let your lovemaking become a slow and graceful dance, so your bodies move harmoniously as if they are melting together. Touch each other with deep respect to honor the body of your lover. Decide that on these special occasions of meditative lovemaking you will try to abstain from orgasm. This will help you to relax deeply together and remain in the moment because you have nothing to achieve except to surrender to the intimacy of the here and now. Do not worry, though, if passion takes over, as you can always practice this method of lovemaking another time. If however, you do introduce meditation into your lovemaking, you will begin to feel its rewards as it brings you into harmony with one another.

To help you create an atmosphere conducive for meditative lovemaking, you can use a blend of frankincense, cedarwood, and rose essential oils in your aromatherapy burner.

AUSTRALIA
Sunspirit Oils Pty. Ltd.
6 Ti-Tree Place
Byron Bay
New South Wales 2481
Tel: 066 856 333

In Essence
3 Abbott Street
Fairfield
Victoria 3078
Tel: 01 497 1411

David Jones Stores
Head Office:
Queen Street
Toowong and Garden City
Queensland 4000
Tel: 02 266 5544

CANADA
Sears Department Stores
Head Office:
Sears of Canada
222 Jarvis Street
Toronto M5B 2B8
Tel: 416 362 1711

Rody & Co. Stockists:
945 Middlefield Road
Unit 14-15
Scarborough
Ontario M1V 5E1
Tel: 416 412 0223

Continental Cosmetics Ltd
Trade Suppliers:
390 Millway Avenue
Concord
Ontario L4K 3V8
Tel: 905 660 0622

FRANCE
Herboristerie
Suppliers:
De La Place Clichy
87 Rue de Amsterdam
75008 - Paris
Tel: 04 874 8332

Herboristerie
du Palais-Royal
11 Rue des Petits-Champs
75001 - Paris
Tel: 04 297 5468

ITALY
Fabrica SRL
Via Cortorine (Angolo via
Valtetrosa)
20123 - Milan
Tel: 02 869 3420

SOUTH AFRICA
Applewoods Int. Ltd.
Distributors:
PO Box 68969
Johannesburg 2120
Tel: 11 442 5328

SWITZERLAND/GERMANY
Covi-Intra AG.
Riedstrasse 5
CH-6330 Cham/
Switzerland
Tel: 41 0 42 422 422

UNITED KINGDOM
Applewoods International Ltd
Heathfield
Newton Abbot
Devon, TQ12 6RY
Tel: 01626 832283

Aromatherapy Products Ltd
(Tisserand)
Newton Road
Hove
East Sussex, BN3 7BA
Tel: 01273 325666

Bodytreats
15 Approach Road
Raynes Park
London SW20 8BA
Tel: 0181 543 763

Fragrant Earth
PO Box 182
Taunton
Somerset, TA1
Tel: 01823 322 566

Swanfleet Oils
93 Fortess Road
London, NW5 1AG
Tel: 0171 267 6717

Culpeper The Herbalist
21 Bruton Street
Berkley Square
London, W1X 7DA
Tel: 0171 629 4559

**UNITED STATES
OF AMERICA**
Applewoods Int. Ltd.
45 Main Street
Westport
Connecticut
CT 06880
Tel: 203 454 2112

Harringtons
325 East Lake Street
Petoskey
Michigan 49770
Tel: 313 882 2419

Avalon Natural Cosmetics, Inc.
1129 Industrial Avenue
Petaluma
California 94952
Tel: 707 769 5120

Body Love Inc.
PO Box 7542
Santa Cruz
California 95061

Quintessence Aromatherapy
PO Box 4996
Boulder
Colorado 80306

INDEX